THE CANCER PATIENT

John J. Dawson

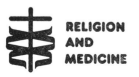

RELIGION AND MEDICINE

Glen W. Davidson, Editor

AUGSBURG PUBLISHING HOUSE
MINNEAPOLIS, MINNESOTA

THE CANCER PATIENT

Scripture quotations unless otherwise noted are from the Revised Standard Version of the Bible, copyright 1946, 1952, and 1971 by the Division of Christian Education of the National Council of Churches.

MANUFACTURED IN THE UNITED STATES OF AMERICA

Contents

To my mother,
whose capacity to love and to die with dignity
taught me how to live.

Foreword

Cancer is called "the modern leprosy" and is for many today's most feared disease. Cancer has not always been the most feared of diseases, nor has chronic disease process been regarded as more loathsome than acute illness, as it is today. In the early days of the Republic, whether it was the expression of Puritan saint or frontier sinner, most people's greatest fear was a quick and unexpected death. Increase Mather, sounding like his clerical colleagues of the 17th century, wrote that if the adult saint were truly in God's grace, the time of death came after an illness in which the sufferer was given a period of torment and testing and an opportunity to repent. Sudden death was an omen of unfaithfulness.

Soon after the Civil War, we find many Americans shifting to the hope that, if Christ's Second Coming were not imminent, quick death was preferable to impaired health. At approximately the same time, public health efforts and laboratory medicine began to discover the causes of infectious diseases —an acute disease process—and Americans seemed to feel more in control of their destiny. By the 1900s, sudden death was not regarded as an omen of unfaithfulness, but a stroke which spared the victim of suffering—a sign interpreted by many faithful as God's blessing. And we can still hear this assumption in the folk theology explaining rapid or sudden death: "at least he didn't have to suffer!"

As chronic disease processes—cancer, arthritis, diabetes, neurological degeneration—became more prominent with better medical control of acute disease processes—heart ailments, infectious diseases, and respiratory failure—many followers of

5

Judaeo-Christian traditions were left without a theology which helped them cope with their suffering. Perhaps no evidence is more striking, or more vicious than the well-meaning saint who informs the cancer sufferer that he or she has the disease "as a result of lack of faith," assuming that suffering is felt in the inverse proportion of one's faith. Those of us who serve in clinical areas repeatedly see such needless pain imposed, all "in the name of the Lord." What a contrast to our 17th century fathers!

This book is added to Augsburg's RELIGION AND MEDICINE SERIES to be of assistance to cancer patients, their families, and health care staff who seek both to cope with the disease process and to interpret it within a theology of life. Its author, John J. Dawson, not only has ministered to thousands of people in similar situations, but has faced the threat of disease in his own family. While his work has been published in technical journals, this is the first time his noteworthy ministry is made available to a general readership.

The author is former Director of the Department of Patient and Family Support Services at the Mountain States Tumor Institute in Boise, Idaho, a position he held for six years. He has been a consultant for other cancer treatment centers in California, Texas, and Montana. At present, he is President of the Patient and Family Support Institute in Boise. He is a member of the Editorial Board of *Death Education: An International Quarterly,* and is a lecturer at Boise State University. He has published articles in *Seminars in Oncology,* and *Proceedings* of the American Association of Clinical Oncologists. He received his education at the University of Maryland and Wesley Theological Seminary. Before becoming a clinician, he served pastorates in Baltimore, Maryland, and Boise, Idaho. He and his wife have three children.

Glen W. Davidson, Ph.D.
Professor and Chairman
Department of Medical Humanities
Southern Illinois University
School of Medicine

A Letter to the Reader

Cancer, to many people, arouses more fear than any other disease. It has become a universal symbol of suffering, pain, and death. Our culture has surrounded cancer with such a mystique that the word itself is never spoken above a whisper by many people. It is as though saying it will cause it. Cancer is bad, but not that bad.

Having cancer often causes patients to have different feelings about themselves and these feelings adversely affect their social interactions. This book has been written to help people in their understanding of the disease, and to assist them in their response to cancer crisis should it come to them or someone they love.

The message of this book could be summarized this way: *Live! Don't Just Survive.* The emphasis here is on quality of life. The first several months after diagnosis, for most cancer patients, are filled with concerns about how long they will live. There is more to life than the postponement of death.

Western thinking has tended to divide the person into three parts, body, mind, and spirit, with medical specialists limited to care for only one of the parts. One's body too often is treated for physical disease with little regard for the impact the mind and spirit may have on the outcome. However, modern health care personnel have an approach to medical treatment in which the patient is regarded as a whole person, not a diseased entity. Health is evaluated in terms of the harmony between body, mind, and spirit, rather than a collection of physical symptoms. The underlying theme of this writing is toward a holistic approach to health care.

7

The data for this book comes primarily from my six years with the Patient and Family Support Team at the Mountain States Tumor Institute. MSTI is a regional outpatient community cancer center in Boise, Idaho. Our staff was engaged in an interdisciplinary approach to the treatment and control of cancer through a program integrating patient care, research, and education.

While the arrangement of words in the text is mine, the basic concepts are the product of the systematic clinical research of a closely knit team dedicated to the improvement of the human condition. The footnote numbers in the text refer to the books listed in the References section at the end of this volume.

I gratefully acknowledge the assistance of my clinical colleagues: Roy E. Buehler, Ph.D., Kenneth Kasner, Ph.D., Cordelia Persigehl, R.N., Sharon Walker, B.S.W., and Julia Ford, R.N., B.S. I must express appreciation to our team of psychosocial research specialists for their methodical and critical evaluation of data: David Monsees, Ph.D., P.K. Tucker, M.S., and Janet Smith, B.S.

We owe a special debt of gratitude to C. Ronald Koons, M.D., and Shirlee Koons, R.N., M.S., whose dedication to the holistic approach in cancer care stimulated and nurtured the concept of our unique patient and family support program. Thanks to Katherine Coursey, B.S., whose pioneering efforts initiated our psychosocial research; and to James K. Luce, M.D., and Charles (Fuzzy) Steuart, M.D., Ph.D., whose constant prodding and critical evaluation got us started and kept us honest. I must also thank Glen W. Davidson, Ph.D., editor, who encouraged me in this writing task and graciously tolerated all my broken deadlines.

My greatest personal debt for the completion of this book is owed to Christine Geier. Her investment in producing a practical guide for those on a journey with cancer is equal to my own. It could not have been accomplished without her constant encouragement, editorial skill, and tireless typing of the manuscript.

Most important in this project are the patients and their families who have taught us all we know about coping with cancer and about quality of life. All the data herein contained has been authenticated in their experience. Only a few of the names are fictitious in order to protect the privacy of individuals. The other names are those of people whose strength and wisdom deserve public recognition. We are indeed honored to be part of such a courageous company.

JOHN J. DAWSON, M.DIV.

1

Cancer: The Modern Leprosy

Disease means different things to different people. To the chronic worrier it poses a constant threat that feeds the fires of his perpetual anxiety. To the healthy person it is an unknown that is never taken seriously—until he gets sick. Then he doesn't know which way to turn or how to cope. To the hypochondriac, disease is an ego trip—especially if he can boast of a minimal illness like his appendicitis that "made medical history."

A major problem with cancer is the erroneous ideas people have regarding the disease and its treatment. The meanings patients attach to cancer can either enhance or impair their self-image and their response to medical treatment. If the patients' unwarranted suspicions are reinforced by the erroneous ideas of others, their emotional stability is threatened and their rehabilitation is compromised.

"The earth stood still the day my doctor told me I had cancer. I remember the walls in my hospital room were a sickly pink. It was an emotional shock to me and my family unlike any other we had experienced. I couldn't believe it—couldn't think straight. At first I didn't want anyone else to know. I couldn't stand the insipid sympathy—being cast as somehow different, separate from the rest of society—like a leper." These words were spoken by a cancer patient sharing his thoughts in a public address just days before his death. It came after years of treatment, remission, recurrence, pain, more treatment, remission, normal living, recurrence, pain, more treatment—and so goes the cycle for him and others as they endure the modern leprosy. I call it leprosy because, to the patients, it often feels like leprosy—an insidious decaying force inside, slowly eating their lives away. I call it leprosy because the patients, like the lepers of biblical days, often find themselves isolated from society, from loved ones, and even from themselves when they discover they have cancer.

Fear of cancer spills over the walls of our concern about physical well-being and infiltrates other areas of life. The capricious nature of cancer, with its unknown quantities, produces an aura of fear around the word itself. The cancer "mystique" has become a symbol of everything evil. The conquest of cancer has become a high priority in our scientific, political, and social life. The average person is frustrated, wondering why we have spent so many billions to send men to the moon when our federal dollars could have been more wisely used to rid our own planet of this evil pestilence. Politicians who support appropriations to cancer research inspire confidence and good will among their constituents. If scientists can discover the cancer cure they will indeed achieve messianic stature.

The Shapes of Anxiety

Just as subconscious fears about the unknown gave terrifying shapes to our childhood nightmares, so uncertainty about cancer gives shape to our adult anxieties. We often repress our anxieties, attempting to evade them. The repression destroys our capacity for rational thinking and our ability to cope. Until we are willing to confront our anxieties and label them, we feel helpless and hopeless. The anxieties churning inside the person who has cancer give shape to meanings he attaches to his adversary.

When Cancer Means Death

To many people cancer is synonymous with death. No other disease brings such an abrupt reminder of our mortality. Some professing Christians like to think they have no fears. But when faced with cancer or another unexpected crisis we all are quickly reminded how real and present fear can be.

Regardless of the depth of our religious experience and convictions, most of us never completely overcome our fear of death. A brilliant young medical school professor, with degrees in Divinity and Psychotherapy, confirms the validity of that statement. While visiting a cancer center on business, he saw a gentleman his own age register as a patient. "An indescribable fear gripped my whole being" he reported, "and I said to myself, 'I thought that I had gotten beyond all that, but I guess I haven't.' " Whether we are rich or poor, highly educated, or fat, dumb, and happy, cancer punctuates our fear of death with incredulous impact.

Perhaps it is loss in death that bothers us; loss of life, loss of significance, separation from loved ones, loss of identity, loss of control, trading the known and tangible for the unseen and unknown. Whatever the reason, the thought of death is so overpowering that we may be tempted to refuse talking about it. Our culture has made death an obscenity. We shield our children from it and scarcely say the word above a whisper, as though saying it might make it happen.

When Cancer Means Pain and Suffering

For many the shape of cancer is pain and suffering. Perhaps death itself is not feared as much as the process of dying. Asked to describe a cancer patient, the average person would probably depict the epitome of suffering and human misery with sunken eyes, gaunt skeletal physique, and sallow complexion.

Because cancer is synonymous with death to many people, they think of a cancer patient as one who has been condemned to a living death. In the minds of many, the tortures of treatment only complicate the terrible suffering. The cancer clinic is visualized as a chamber of horrors. Even though we speak of the remarkable advances of medical science, many see the cancer specialist as a mad scientist engaged in unethical use of human guinea pigs for some futile experimentation. We are fearful that if the disease doesn't get us, the treatment will.

When Cancer Means Being Contaminated

Cancer is often thought of as a contaminating disease—the patient is contaminated and contaminates everyone he touches. I once knew a clergyman who went straight to the washroom after visiting a cancer patient in the hospital. Some patients get the feeling they should wear surgical masks and walk though town crying, "Unclean! Unclean!"

In our society, we tend to think of people with heart conditions as hardworking, straight shooting, clean-cut American individualists. For some strange reason a heart condition to some people is a status symbol. A malignancy, on the other hand, stimulates an entirely different reaction. It is a disease with a different value. Cancer patients are pitied. Most of us can't look them in the eye, let alone converse with them. Perhaps it is because they symbolize to us that slender thread of mortality which ties us to life. One of the most difficult initial adjustments for many patients with cancer results from being relegated to this different status of human existence.

When Cancer Means Being Ostracized

Some patients report that friends avoid them because of their fear that cancer is catching. One patient relates that her neighbor did not visit her for six months following cancer surgery. "I am sorry I didn't visit you sooner," she apologized. "I guess after all this time it's safe now." This lady's lack of sensitivity was exceeded only by her ignorance about cancer. But ostracism does not mean only losing friends. Some patients lose their job once the employer hears of the diagnosis. Patients who are school age children sometimes are denied the opportunity to return to their classroom. Some well-meaning friends can stimulate guilt and ostracism by saying things like, "I can't believe that you, of all people, have *cancer*. If only you could have detected it sooner." Small wonder that having cancer to many patients also means being ostracized.

When Cancer Means Being Made Dependent

The fear of not being able to care for oneself and of becoming completely dependent upon others is demeaning and unacceptable for most of us. For some patients just the diagnosis of cancer is enough to stimulate dependency. With progression of the disease restrictions are made on the patients' physical and mental activity. Often their freedom for making decisions is usurped by the family or is surrendered by the patients themselves.

When Cancer Means Being Abandoned

There is a vast difference between solitude and loneliness. All people need time apart from the world to collect their thoughts and gain a better perspective. Such solitude is usually self-imposed and a welcome relief from the helter-skelter routine. Time apart for spiritual reflection is necessary to refresh the mind and help one cope with the stresses of everyday living.

Solitude is elected, loneliness is inflicted. We are social beings and need the support of other people. We simply cannot live without it. Newborn babies who have been abandoned in the hospital wither and die unless someone becomes a surrogate mother, providing human warmth and affection. Some primitive societies still abandon the weak and elderly who cannot contribute to the general welfare of the community. The loneliness inflicted on these individuals hastens their death.

For many, having cancer means receiving a life sentence to solitary confinement. They feel estranged and alone—even in a crowd. The nuances of discomfort experienced by others in their presence raise serious questions for patients. "If they are uncomfortable now, how will they feel if my illness grows worse? Will they stay around or leave me?" Dying alone in a foul-smelling nursing home represents for most people the worst of all possible fates. Newly diagnosed cancer patients may project that fate for themselves. Fear of illness and death is threatening. Fear of being ill and dying alone is intolerable.

When Anxieties Are Confirmed

For our purposes in this text I define anxiety as unfocused suspicion. The anxieties experienced by newly diagnosed patients may be out of proportion with reality, but they are real to them and can't be waved away with a magic wand—or even a word of prayer. The initial effect of a cancer diagnosis on human relationships tends to confirm suspicions of the patient.

This factor is apparent even in childhood cancer. Pediatric patients suddenly live in a world of specialized people and procedures. They are the objects of intense concern and increased attention from their parents. They are set apart from their siblings. They often respond with jealousy, hostility, and confusion. Their confusion arises from their ambivalence. They feel sympathy and jealousy simultaneously. Parents and other adults often experience the same feelings. Parents love their children. The abundance of attention begins to spoil them. When they behave accordingly, their hostility is aroused. The anger, frustration, and sympathy are in conflict. How does one discipline a dying child—especially when that child is your own?

Sometimes this same process erodes the relationship between husband and wife. Both patient and spouse "protect" each other by not expressing their feelings. The resulting sense of isolation stimulates ambivalence. The relationship is threatened, and the patient's suspicions are confirmed. Loss of job is another experience which tends to confirm the patient's anxieties regarding ostracism, dependency, and abandonment. Physical constraints of the illness may precipitate occupational disability. Employers' response to the diagnosis of cancer by termination of the patient as a poor risk is not uncommon. This phenomenon has been observed in studies conducted by the National Cancer Institute and has been the subject of a network television documentary.

Society's reaction to the cancer patient is often primitive in its fear, suspicion, and insensitivity. Every patient is painfully aware of the friends who no longer come around, or those who do but don't know what to say. Even medical personnel, attempting to be empathetic, often reinforce anxiety. One patient reports the manner in which she was told of her diagnosis:

> They put my husband and me in a small examining room. After waiting a long time, both physicians came in. I could tell by the expressions on their faces they had bad news. They looked at the floor and then at each other. Finally, one said, "Mrs. Simpson, I don't want to frighten you, but . . . you have cancer." Now really, there is nothing more frightening than a doctor who says he doesn't want to frighten you. These men were cancer specialists having all that trouble giving a diagnosis. It's no wonder general practitioners are so afraid of their cancer patients!

Another patient reported, "I wish my doctor could look me in the eye and say, 'Frank, you have cancer.' Instead he evades direct eye contact and makes me feel as though I had syphilis or leprosy or some other social disease."

Still another patient stated, "On my first trip to the cancer center I thought to myself, 'I don't belong here. I'm not a leper!' Suddenly I realized—I am one of them."

These prevalent societal reactions to cancer serve to reinforce the patients' new sensitivities that they are "different," and confirm their suspicions regarding the modern leprosy. A well-known celebrity suffering from cancer decided to keep her diagnosis secret. She hired a secretary her own size who did all her personal shopping so that not even clothing salesclerks would know she'd had a mastectomy.

Getting a Better Perspective

Although cancer can be a serious life-threatening illness, it is not always the frightening adversary many imagine. Most of the meanings attached to cancer that are listed in this chapter are exaggerated or erroneous. Not everyone who has the disease dies of it, but every cancer patient must confront the fear of death. That confrontation can help set more appropriate life priorities and realistic goals. When we accept our own finiteness we may take life more seriously, and ourselves less seriously. We can allow ourselves the freedom to fail. Freedom to fail stimulates freedom to venture. We can never achieve true fulfillment in life until we are free to fail. This book is based on the ventures and victories of hundreds of people whose journey with cancer brought that freedom.

Suffering and pain is usually part of an experience with cancer, but not always. Given the current state of medical arts and seeing pain in proper perspective can minimize suffering, if not completely alleviate it.

Cancer need not be the modern leprosy. Ignorance about the disease and treatment has given rise to the mythical suspicions that comprise the cancer mystique. The erroneous meanings we attach to cancer can be destructive. Separating fact from fantasy helps us to know what to expect. Knowing what to expect gives rise to a positive coping stategy.

Many people have learned, through their experience with cancer, that although we cannot always change the circumstances life has presented us, we can make a positive change in our response to those circumstances. That change can mean the difference between victory or defeat. Mike Smith, a 21-year-old man with Hodgkin's disease, tells how he decided to win:

> looming before me like the open jaws
> of a monster,
> whose appetite will never be satisfied.
> I cannot penetrate the shadows,
> only try to live with them.
> the choice is mine,
> slide to my oblivion or maybe, just maybe,
> to overcome.
> neither will come easy.
> one long leap would do it,
> but what would it prove?
> only that I couldn't handle it
> and I have been reminded of that fact
> all of my life.
> they might be proven wrong.
> the other road is no easier.
> to others,
> it is the natural choice,
> but they don't have to walk it,
> I do.
> If I fail I will have to pick it up again.
> past mistakes cannot be corrected
> but neither can they be forgotten.
> the victories must come from day to day.
> If they do not,
> the final one will never be achieved.

The degree of ostracism, dependency, and abandonment people with cancer may experience depends, in large measure, upon themselves and their response to their illness. Coping with the physical, emotional, and social adjustments of cancer can present patients with a formidable set of anxieties. They must learn to be realistic about their suspicions, work through them, and help those who want to "help," but don't know what to say or what to do. It can be done. We begin by separating fact from fantasy. Then we turn unfocused suspicions into identified fears that can be confronted. Next we develop a coping strategy that builds upon small daily victories to achieve the final one. Cancer need not be the end. It can be a new beginning.

2

What Is Cancer?
Separating Fact
from Fantasy

What is cancer? How is it caused—
food additives, poor diet, pollution
of the environment, personal living habits? How is it
treated? Can it be cured? Cancer is a disease that has been
around for a long time and is currently on the increase. It
is projected that one person in four will be directly affected
by it next year. Only heart disease claims more lives than
cancer.

As we have seen in the previous chapter, cancer precipitates a remarkable degree of emotional responses. An essential aspect of adequate coping with cancer is getting the facts.
Sufficient knowledge and understanding of this disease may
enable us to maintain a degree of emotional equanimity when
faced with a personal cancer crisis. Let us first consider the
nature of the disease as illness.

The Case of the Rebellious Cell (What Is Cancer?)

The study of the human cell structure is like a fascinating
journey to the heart of the universe. Right on target was the
psalmist who observed "my body is fearfully and wonder-
fully made." The tiny cells which constitute more than 120

21

different forms of tissue in the human body must live in harmony in order for the individual to enjoy a healthy life. Each cell has its own microcosmic anatomy with indwelling systems that regulate its nutrient, growth, reproduction and activity. If one of the cell's subsystems goes awry it can get sick and die. If it fails to compute properly a message governing its function, the cell may deviate from its intended purpose and create a serious threat to the life of the body it inhabits.

Cancer occurs when one cell decides to deviate from the purpose and function for which it was created. It begins to divide and grow in an uncontrolled manner. Sometimes the immune responses of the body, like resident policemen, can put down this cellular rebellion. It is generally believed that most people experience such premalignant conditions several times during their life span. However, if the malignancy goes unchecked it will become invasive, destructive, and ultimately threaten the life of the individual. It is difficult to conceive that one very tiny cell can wreak such havoc in a living organism. It is difficult to understand how such a tiny deviation could culminate in such personal and social devastation. The destructive potential unleashed by a rebellious cell in the human body is an awesome phenomenon to ponder.

If Only the Whole Truth Were Known (What Causes Cancer?)

Cancer is not one, but many diseases. Its name is Legion. Malignancies can occur in any type of tissue in the human body. The word *cancer* is an umbrella title for more than 120 different forms of malignancy. The researcher seeking a cause and the physician determining a treatment cannot consider a singular problem and solution, but are faced with a complexity of diseases compounded by a variety of symptoms.

What causes a normal cell to become malignant is only

partially understood. There seem to be several causative factors. One known factor is exposure to chemicals (such as those present in tobacco smoke) that stimulate malignancy in normal cells. These chemicals damage the normal cells by making them more susceptible to the development of cancer. A number of these cancer-producing chemicals, known as carcinogens, have been identified. Some are present in the atmosphere as a result of industrial pollution. Some have been identified in food processing, such as cyclamates. There are many other suspected carcinogens that have not been thoroughly studied.

Another factor in the cause of cancer may be viruses which have been demonstrated to cause malignancies in lower animals, such as mice and rats. However, there is no strong evidence to substantiate that viruses cause cancer, or that cancer is an infectious or contagious disease.

Although there may be some genetic predisposition in some cells to cancer, there is no conclusive evidence that cancer is hereditary. Genetic implications of cancer are difficult to study in humans because of our longevity. What is true in laboratory studies for the prolific fruit fly, with his short life span, may not apply to humans. While some forms of cancer seem to run in some families, there is nothing conclusive upon which to base a solid theory.

It is generally agreed among scientists that there is no single cause, but a combination of factors occurring simultaneously to produce malignancies. To control the environment in such a way as to eliminate all carcinogens would be like trying to hold back the tide with a broom. Curing a cancer that has a running start has not proven effective. Early diagnosis is currently the best assurance of control of cancer. However, to date there are no effective means of early detection for the most deadly forms of malignancies. Many scientists believe that effective cancer control will ultimately be achieved by discovering how to control the rebellious cell, not by improved treatment methods.

The Insidious Traveler
(How Cancers Grow and Spread)

Once the malignant changes occur, the cell begins to grow out of control. Initially the cellular formations are microscopic. Approximately one million tightly packed cells occupy a space equivalent to the head of a pin. By the time a cancer is detectable, it may have grown to several billion cells. All tumors are the result of an uncontrolled growth of cells, but not all tumors are malignant. Benign tumors remain localized. Malignant tumors slough off cells which can travel to other areas of the body and begin to grow again. These malignant cells can travel through the lymph channels to the lymph nodes and, via the blood vessels, throughout the entire body. If the new environment is favorable to these cells they will grow and multiply. Common places for this growth are the bone marrow, liver, and lungs. This process is called metastasis.

A primary tumor may remain small and produce no adverse symptoms. It may shed cells into the bloodstream for many years before one of the cells finds an environment conducive to its growth. An individual may have an undetected malignancy for years. His cancer may be discovered only when the metastatic lesion begins to grow and produce symptoms. If the primary tumor remains small and cannot be discovered, adequate control of the disease is usually impossible.

Cancer is, indeed, an insidious and capricious traveler.

Cancer as a Chronic Disease

Not everyone who has cancer dies of it. Two out of every six patients are cured. Three out of six will die because of lack of medical knowledge and ability to cure them. One will die simply because of failure to get to the doctor in time. All forms of cancer could be cured if diagnosed soon enough.

Unfortunately, by the time most cancers become symptomatic they have grown too large to be controlled and have metastasized.

Due to the nature of the malignant process it is possible for a single sequestered cell to lie dormant for years before beginning to grow again. Therefore, even though the primary tumor has been removed the cancer may begin to grow again months or years later. For this reason, except for the few types of malignancies that can be cured, cancer must be considered a chronic rather than acute illness. The implication for patients is that they will probably have to live with malignancy the rest of their lives. So often after surgery the physicians declare they "got it all," meaning all they saw. However, it is the remaining microscopic malignant cell that may begin to grow again and threaten the individual's health and life. The recurrence of cancer strikes most patients with an exceedingly powerful impact.

The Hopeful Side of Cancer

There are some hopeful signs regarding cancer cure. Death from cervical cancer will probably be obliterated in our lifetime. Cervical cancer is now 80% curable. It is nearly 100% curable when caught in its earliest stages. Early diagnosis facilitated by the Pap Smear has made this advance possible. While cancer of the cervix is easily detectable by this method, malignancies of the uterus and ovaries must be detected by thorough pelvic examination. Women should receive a complete gynecological examination at least once a year.

As recently as six years ago, Hodgkin's Disease was considered an incurable form of cancer. Today, thirty out of every hundred cases of Hodgkin's Disease can be cured. When caught in its earliest stages it is 95% curable. Even some forms of leukemia, through new drugs and experimental procedures such as bone marrow transplant, are being cured. Even though the cure rate for breast cancer is no better than it was 50 years ago, survival rates have been significantly increased by advanced methods of treatment.

The word cure must be cautiously applied to cancer. When malignancies are controlled for long periods of time, physicians often refer to five or ten year cures. Perhaps a more accurate term is *remission*. A remission from cancer is achieved when there is no clinical evidence of malignancy following a course of treatment. Sequestered cells may exist somewhere in the body, but are too small to be detected. The patient is safe until those cells begin to grow again.

Even though most forms of cancer cannot be cured, many can be significantly controlled for long periods of time. Many cancer patients achieve long term remissions up to 25 years. Some patients may die of a nonmalignant condition before the sequestered cells begin to grow again. For this reason many scientists now classify cancer as a chronic rather than a terminal illness. Most chronic illnesses are not curable. Many of these diseases can be arrested and controlled, but never cured. Many people with cancer, however, are completely cured.

Cancer as Visualized Fear

For many, the fear of cancer is the essence of the disease. That is, visualization of fear itself becomes for the individual the reality of the illness. We have already listed anxieties that are usually stimulated by a cancer diagnosis.

Approximately two-thirds of all people with cancer will die from the disease. Most of those individuals, through advanced methods of treatment, can gain adequate control over the disease and achieve increased longevity and quality of life.

Appropriate confrontation with the probability of death as a result of a cancer diagnosis is essential for both patient and family. While death is a realistic possibility, it must be seen in perspective. Even though we know intellectually that death is inevitable, at the emotional level most of us would do almost anything to escape it. Polls continue to confirm that most people, when they die, want to die instantly. It has not always been that way, nor is it in all cultures today. Some would prefer "time to prepare myself and my family." Most patients with cancer have that opportunity. For a very helpful approach to death see another book in this series, *Living with Dying,* by Dr. Glen W. Davidson.

Fear of pain and suffering is the second most prevalent fear. Fear of suffering and death often deters people from reporting symptoms to a physician. If a malignancy is indeed present, delay of treatment will lead to fears confirmed! Early diagnosis is the best assurance against suffering and death from cancer. Today the goal of medical therapy, when cure is not possible, is alleviation of pain by controlling tumor growth. One cancer specialist says that only about one-third of patients with cancer have significant pain. With available analgesics, long acting drugs, such as methadone, and cognitive conditioning, adequate pain control for all patients is possible.

Fear that cancer is hereditary or contagious is another prevalent concern. Although some studies have indicated the possibility of an inherent genetic predisposition toward cancer and that particles of viruses have been isolated in malignant cells, there is no conclusive evidence that cancer is either hereditary or contagious. Even if the risk of infectious transmission of cancer does exist, it is apparently very low.

Cancer is indeed a serious illness which can cause suffering and death. There are enough factors inherent in this capricious disease to stimulate valid concerns, without arousing disproportionate fears through misconceptions regarding cancer and its treatment. Direct confrontation of reality is often less threatening than partial understanding combined with strong imagination. Essential to an adequate approach to the cancer crisis is the process of separating valid fears from misconceptions. When all the known facts have been gathered, workable alternatives can be formulated and rational choices can be made.

Once a cancer is diagnosed, there are many medical alternatives for the patient. Sometimes only one of several medical possibilities is the appropriate treatment. A multidisciplinary approach is the preferred treatment today. We will now explore the medical options for the patient with cancer.

A Clear Cut Decision (Surgery)

Once a cancer is diagnosed the most obvious approach is surgical removal. However, sometimes tumors are attached to vital organs or blood vessels rendering surgery impossible without undue threat to the life of the patient. Even when all gross disease (that which can be seen with the naked eye) can be removed, the probability of remaining microscopic cells presents a clear and present threat to the patient. Therefore, further treatment is often appropriate after surgery.

Most surgical procedures for cancer are extensive, though some are more radical than others. These procedures often alter the body image and require considerable adjustment in life-style. For example, many women feel sexually inadequate and unappealing following radical mastectomy.

One of the most prevalent forms of cancer surgery is the mastectomy for malignancies of the breast. There are three forms of breast surgery depending on the extent of the malignancy:

1. *Simple Mastectomy* in which only the breast is removed.
2. *Modified Radical* in which the breast and adjacent lymph nodes are removed.
3. *Radical Mastectomy* in which the breast, the pectoral muscle which lies under the breast, and the lymph nodes which lie behind the breast between the arm and the chest are removed.

Some surgeons choose the procedure in which they have the most training and experience. Surgeons well versed in an interdisciplinary approach to cancer treatment are well aware of the capabilities of post operative radiation and chemotherapy and perform the minimum surgery for the maximum assurance of control of the malignancy.

Some surgeons advocate the lumpectomy in which only the tumor is removed leaving the breast intact. Subcutaneous mastectomy is another recent modification of breast surgery. This procedure removes all glandular tissue from the breast, preserving the outer layer of flesh with immediate implantation of a breast prosthesis.

About 90% of all lumps discovered in the breast are not malignant. Most surgeons explain, prior to surgery, that the lump will be removed and examined under a microscope while the patient is under anesthesia. If it is malignant, the appropriate surgery will be performed immediately. An alternate, perhaps preferable method is to have the lump taken out and examined. If it is cancer, a mastectomy can then be done a few days later. This is called a two-stage operative procedure and is one advocated by many physicians. A consent form must be signed by the patient before anything is done.

For many women, just the prospect of having cancer is so threatening that the emotional reaction short-circuits the mental processes preventing all the information regarding surgery from being assimilated. Women faced with the possibility of breast surgery should request a full explanation of all surgical options from their physician. They should feel free to ask for a repeat explanation and request time to think about it. If there is still a reasonable doubt concerning alternatives, a second opinion from a surgeon who is not heavily committed to a specific procedure should be sought.

For many women a mastectomy is no great trauma. They feel the loss of a breast is a fair trade for control of a life-threatening malignancy, and spend a relatively short time grieving the loss. The Reach For Recovery Program sponsored by the American Cancer Society is a valuable resource for the mastectomy patient. This volunteer corps of fellow patients, upon recommendation of the surgeon, visit new patients prior to their release from the hospital. They provide emotional support and specific instructions for physical rehabilitation.

Colectomy is another prevalent form of cancer surgery in which the cancer along with a piece of the colon is removed. In doing this operation, the surgeon may have to make a colostomy, either temporarily or permanently. A colostomy is the result when the bowel end is brought through the skin of the abdomen and sutured into place. This results in defecation through an opening in the abdomen. Adjustment to this surgery is often repulsive and denigrating to the patient and his spouse.

The initial physical and emotional trauma of a colostomy can be very disturbing to the patient. However, by the time he is discharged from the hospital his abdominal opening is no longer swollen and unsightly. He has received adequate instruction and experience in ostomy care. He may have received a visitor from the American Cancer Society's local Ostomy Club. The membership of this club is comprised of ostomy patients and their spouses. They provide mutual emotional support and shared technique in ostomy care.

With established eating patterns and adequate care of the ostomy most people can regulate its function. They enjoy normal physical activity with little or no social embarrassment. One patient quipped, "My ostomy is a matter of convenience. I don't need to make all of those rest stops on long trips anymore."

These are only two types of cancer surgery. This modality has become highly specialized. Patients facing surgery should be aware of the surgeon's specialty and be very clear in understanding all options of a particular type of cancer surgery. Do not be timid in asking for repeat explanations.

Spot Checkmate (Radiation)

Radiation therapy is often used to eliminate microscopic cancer cells remaining at the surgical site. Radiation therapy uses penetrating ionizing rays (x-rays) for the treatment of cancer and tumors. It is used primarily in the treatment of cancer: Occasionally noncancerous tumors are also treated.

Radiation is most effective in treating localized malignancies. Many cancers may be likened to a weed growing in a garden. Such weeds can be managed by digging them up (surgical removal) or treating them with local concentration of weed killer (radiation therapy).

The basic effects of radiation therapy are those of destroying the ability of the cells to multiply and grow. This process takes place in tumor cells and in normal tissue cells alike. However, radiation is used when the tumor cells are more sensitive than the surrounding normal tissue and the normal cells have the ability to repair the damage done by the radiation. Accurate planning of the treatment insures that all the tumor is treated, but that the beam of radiation passes through as little normal tissue as possible. Application of radiation in small divided doses over a prolonged period of time increases the injury to the tumor cells with less injury to the normal tissue. Different forms of radiation are appropriately used to treat various malignancies.

Skin cancers are generally treated with x-ray. The x-ray beam delivers the intensity of its radiation to the surface of the skin and is most effective with superficial malignancies. Most skin cancers are cured with 30 to 40 treatments. Treatments last only a few minutes and are generally administered once a day five days a week.

In certain circumstances, it is desirable to place radioactive sources directly into the tumor site. In years past, radium was the most frequently used material. With the dawning of the atomic age, most radium has been replaced by man-made radioactive materials which perform the same function as radium but usually with greater safety. These radioactive materials may be placed into the tumor in the form of needles or capsules, or may be applied against the tumor in some type of applicator. The patients receiving radioactive implants must be hospitalized in a private room in order not to expose others unduly to the radiation. Once the radioactive sources are removed there is no residual radioactivity left in the body. Radiation implants are used most prevalently in the treatment of cervical and uterine cancer.

Internal tumors require high energy radiation penetrating more deeply into the body. One such high energy source of radiation comes from cobalt. Because radioactive cobalt delivers the intensity of its radiation at a deeper level than x-ray, tumors can be treated with little or no injury to the skin or surface tissues.

The linear accelerator is a radiation machine which manufactures its own more powerful and precise beam of radiation. Linear acceleration is currently the most advanced method of radiation therapy.

There are many prevalent misconceptions regarding radiation therapy and its side effects. There is no pain connected with radiation treatment. Hair loss occurs only in the area that is treated. Fatigue is the most common side effect of radiation, and is easily controlled with proper diet and increased rest. Sometimes skin irritation results from radiation. Most side effects of radiation therapy subside within three weeks after treatment is completed. Excessive amounts of radiation can cause delayed reactions years after treatment. However, the qualified radiation therapist plans treatment so that the benefits far exceed the possible or potential side effects.

For some forms of cancer, radiation is the primary source of treatment through which cure can be achieved. It is most often used in conjunction with other forms of treatment. Radiation is a well established method of treatment having been in use for many years. Its limits have been delineated and most tumors are affected by it.

A Search and Destroy Strategy (Chemotherapy)

When malignant tumors have metastasized widely throughout the body, or in forms of cancer not manifesting themselves in solid tumors, the disease is systemic. In these situations surgery or localized radiation therapy are inappropriate and insufficient to control the malignancy. When a few isolated dandelions appear in a lawn they can be pulled up or destroyed by spot weed killer. When the whole lawn is covered with dandelions it is necessary to spray the entire surface with weed killer. Likewise, when cancer has seeded itself throughout the body, localized treatment is ineffective. Chemicals which are known to be toxic to specific kinds of tumors are then used since they are carried by the blood to all body tissues. When given in the vein or by mouth the chemicals spread throughout the body and attack cancer cells.

Chemotherapy is usually used against cancers which have spread to other tissues and those tumors which are not expected to respond to other kinds of treatment. There are some conditions in which chemotherapy is the only effective treatment. In several of these diseases chemotherapy can cure these patients. Examples include: acute leukemia in children, some forms of Hodgkin's Disease, tumors of the womb and testicles. The way in which chemotherapy works is to stop the growth and division of malignant cells. Some normal cells have rapid growth and division. These cells are also frequently harmed by chemotherapy, but recover faster than cancer cells.

Chemicals usually do not kill all the cancer cells. When they do work, the response may be temporary. This is because the cells which are not killed become resistent to the chemicals and the cancer starts to grow again. When this happens the physician usually stops treatment with the drug or drug combinations and employs a different treatment.

As treatment methods and chemicals improve, more patients are being cured of their cancer with chemotherapy. The number of drugs used in cancer treatment is growing. One class of drugs called Antimetabolites interferes with the cells' ability to replicate genes. Two frequently used Antimetabolites are 5-Fluorouracil (5-FU) and Methotrexate. They are ordinarily given by vein and are frequently used in combination with other drugs. Another group of drugs is known as Alkylating Agents because of their chemical actions. Examples of these drugs are Cytoxan^R, and Leukeran^R. They can be given by mouth or vein depending on the type of disease and the plan for treatment. Another group of drugs is called the antitumor antibiotics because they are made from molds like penicillin. Some of these are very new and some are still under investigation. Examples of antibiotics are Dactinomycin and Adriamycin.

Another group, the Vinca Alkaloids, are made from the periwinkle plant. Examples of these are Vincristine and Vinblastine. They are very commonly used in combination with other drugs because they kill tumor cells in a different way and add to the cell killing ability of the other drugs.

Chemotherapy is not always successful. It may be that the cancer cells are resistent to the drug from the beginning of treatment or they may later become resistent. Although research is being conducted to determine before treatment whether the patient will respond, no certain method has been developed. At present the best way to test effectiveness is by treatment.

All drugs have side effects. Commonly encountered side effects of cancer drugs are numbness and tingling in the fingers, hair loss, mouth ulcers, nausea and vomiting. These side effects are usually caused because of the action of the chemicals against the rapidly dividing cells in the hair follicles and sensitive epithelial cells lining the mouth and stomach. Nausea and vomiting can usually be controlled by antinausea drugs. Patients experiencing hair loss usually regain a full head of hair when treatment is terminated. Some patients regain their hair during the course of treatment. Obviously, as with all treatments that have the possibility of considerable benefits, there is usually some risk involved. The attending cancer specialist usually takes considerable time in explaining the medical alternatives open to the cancer patient.

Fighting Fire with Fire (Immunotherapy)

A fourth medical alternative employed in the treatment of cancer is immunotherapy. The purpose of this method is to stimulate the body's immune response in order to put down the rebellion of malignant cells. The development of vaccines have been effective in such dread diseases as tuberculosis, smallpox and polio. Because of the complexity of cancer a single vaccine for its many different forms is not a realistic hope. The search for such a vaccine began at the turn of the century. Lack of success lead to lack of funds and interest on the part of scientists. With the discovery of some drugs that seem to be effective with certain forms of cancer there is renewed interest in the field of immunotherapy. Even though this is a relatively undeveloped area, many scientists think that it holds the promise of future cancer control. Control of individual immune responses may be a more probable preventive approach than attempting total control of the environment.

The Fifth Dimension (Emotional Support)

The emotional trauma of a cancer diagnosis may be as threatening to both the patient and the family as the physiological aspects of this disease. An insidiously destructive disease that threatens rapid degeneration, radical treatment procedures, long term suffering and ultimate death can be most devastating to one's sense of personal identity. How does one come to grips internally with the stark reality of the consequences of a cancer diagnosis? How does it effect one's thoughts about oneself, one's present involvements, one's hopes and dreams for the future? How does one approach his or her spouse with the implications of sweeping changes in life-style, or even termination of their relationship? How does one keep cool under stress like that? How does the family breadwinner cope with early disability retirement with its threat of financial and emotional dependency? How does the spouse cope with changing to the role of breadwinner? What does a young mother say to her children when faced with the possibility that she will not live to see them come of age?

What do parents say to their child stricken with cancer who is old enough to feel pain and fear medical procedures, but too young to understand the stark realities of life and death? How do they explain it all to brothers and sisters of the ill child? What are the feelings of the siblings toward the patient, toward the parents, and about themselves?

What about the threat of loss to a dependent senior citizen whose spouse is a cancer victim? Should we assume that because they have lived a long life elderly people should not fear illness and death? Does their age and maturity magically lighten the burden of grief and loneliness?

These are questions for which answers cannot be found in test tubes or computers. In an age of technological advancement and medical specialization it is easier to stick stethoscopes in our ears and listen to heart beats instead of heart throbs. Yet these are questions that represent the essence of meaning and purpose for all of us. Preoccupation with the technological function of the human organism can give us more longevity to ponder these questions, but it cannot give us the answers. Science is a servant, not a savior.

"I am so jittery and shaky I can't even get a job. It's a life of hell. Liquor is the best answer," wrote a Midwestern housewife whose husband and 18-year-old son both died of cancer within two years.

A New England attorney said that the experience of watching his 10-year-old daughter die of leukemia "is still vivid and unreal" four years later. "I still lay awake nights thinking about her and have fits of depression which are obvious around the holidays. My wife and I have ulcers as a result of the years of waiting and watching 'nothing serious.' "

A study at Stanford University Medical Center shows the reaction of the Midwestern housewife and New England attorney are typical. Dr. David M. Kaplan, an expert in

Psychiatric Social Work has studied forty families shortly after the death of a leukemia patient and the study showed massive emotional and physical health problems among the mourners.

Physically, 90 percent of the families had at least one member who later became ill. Almost as many reported that some members suffered from "morbid grief reactions": They had problems working, going to school, and taking care of the house. Thirty-five percent of the families had one member in psychiatric treatment after the death and forty percent reported someone in the family had developed a drinking problem.

The death also hurt the parents' relationship with their other children, and in seventy percent of the families, aggravated marital problems. The death was blamed for divorce in two families and separations in seven families.

Ironically, new treatment methods that keep cancer patients alive longer often exacerbate the emotional problems that they and their families face.

"The multiple crises in cancer exhausts the parents emotionally," said Kaplan, "and often leads to the feelings that they wish the child would die." Dr. Kaplan asserts that detecting the emotional problems clearly is as important to the patient's successful treatment as the early detection is to medical treatment.

Physicians are now beginning to recognize this. Dr. LaSalle d'Lefall of Howard University School of Medicine said he has learned from his patients how his unconscious feelings affect their care. One breast cancer patient, for example, noted that the doctor did not spend as much time with her as he did with other patients. Moreover, he ascribed her weakening condition to the spread of cancer. When he later found out that it was due to a treatable and unrelated chemical imbalance, he said, "I wasn't doing my job as a doctor." Public attitudes toward cancer were formed at a time when it was considered a hopeless disease, he said, and the strong emotional fear it generates is due to the feeling that it always involves pain, helplessness, and hopelessness. "When people think about cancer, they think of the worst kind of cancer that anyone they knew ever had."

Dr. Jerome W. Yates of the University of Vermont College of Medicine said recently treatment advances are changing the public conception of cancer. While it still kills 370,000 Americans a year, people are living normal lives for longer times with the disease and some forms of cancer are considered curable.

No comprehensive medical care plan can exclude the psychological and social implications of physical illness. The intensity of individual and cultural reactions to the cancer mystique demands special attention to these factors when treating cancer patients and their families. The result of a family's experience with cancer can be emotionally, vocationally, and financially devastating.

In its frantic quest for perpetual youth, intellectual supremacy and technological excellence, our generation has seen the empathetic family physician replaced by a monolithic medical machine. The health care professions are beginning to realize how impersonal and dehumanizing our technology has become. There is a rapidly growing interest in investigating the inclusion in medical treatment planning of psychosocial factors and their effect on response to medical therapy. Technology is sterile, but medical technologists desire to be humane. Most medical centers are now expanding their multidisciplinary emphasis to include the psychosocial dimension of patient care.

The implications of this renewed interest in the human condition has broad implications for us as individuals and for society in general. The remainder of this book will address itself to the nonmedical human needs of cancer victims. Its rationale is an outgrowth of the collective experience of clinicians and patients alike who are learning to cope with the cancer experience.

3

Is the Body
the Servant
of the Mind?

To what extent can the mind affect the physiological processes of the body? Can we *think* ourselves into illness? If so, can we *will* ourselves well? That is possible with tension headaches and upset stomach from stress and anxiety, but is it possible with a more serious illness? Convincing evidence to the affirmative is increasing. If the evidence is true, what about faith healing? What is the significance of all this to people coping with cancer? There are definite answers to some of these questions and some helpful guidelines in areas not so well defined.

It must be emphasized that critical thinking and insistence on empirical data are prerequisite to such an exploration. Otherwise, wishful thinking, rumor and fantasy will distort our perspective with gross inaccuracy. This is an area of human experience which has fascinated both the scholarly and unschooled since the beginning of human history. Much that has come from both quarters can be dismissed as unreliable and invalid speculation, often biased by erroneous presuppositions and motivated by a desire to rationalize longstanding dogma. It is not the intent of this chapter to explore the areas of metaphysics or psychic phenomenon, but to consider empirical data from human experience in order to bring some degree of illumination to those perplexed by chronic or life threatening illness.

Correlation of Phychological Stress to Physical Illness

Let us first consider some evidence from systematic research and clinical experience which demonstrates the impact of the mind on body chemistry. Medical science has already substantiated the fact that anxiety and tension can and do affect physiological response. Some diseases such as peptic ulcer, colitis and some forms of heart disease can be directly attributed to stress. Scientists now suspect that some infectious and autoimmune diseases may be attributed to stress. Among these are infectious mononucleosis and arthritis.

Doctors Meyer Friedman and Ray Rosenman have defined the Type A and B personalities and their correlation to heart disease.[5] The Type A personality is the person committed to high achievement. Compulsive in his activities, often beginning another project before his first is completed, he keeps an excessively busy schedule and is generally aggressive. He is regarded as a high risk candidate for coronary disease.

The Type B personality, by contrast, is quiet, methodical, and generally passive. He has no great aspirations for fame, fortune or success. He paces himself and seldom physically overexerts. He is not generally prone to heart disease. Studies in the role of stress in physical illness indicate that the person who rallies to a cause, becomes overly excited at a game, or is easily emotionally stimulated in religious activity is most likely to have physical illness precipitated by stress. Conversely, people who are more placid, do not tend to be impetuous in action or erratic in behavior and are more rational than impetuous in decision-making are less prone to stress-produced and psychosomatic illnesses.

There is strong clinical evidence that intense emotional response to certain situations can cause sudden death. As far back as written records exist, people are described as dying suddenly while in the throes of fear, rage, grief, humiliation, or joy, a fate often believed by the devout to be sanctioned by divine edict. Thus the Bible tells us that when Ananias was charged by Peter, "You have not lied to men, but to God!" he fell down dead. So did his wife, Sapphira, when told, "Hark, the feet of those that have buried your husband are at the door, and they will carry you out" (Acts 5:4, 9).

As recent as May, 1971 the *Annals of Internal Medicine* reported a study in rapid death from psychological distress.[20] The common denominators in the deaths of 170 persons were overwhelming excitation, loss of control, and giving up. The study demonstrates strong evidence of high correlation between psychological stress and sudden death.

There is little question that emotional response has a significant effect on physiological processes. Some of the most definitive research in physiological response to anxiety produced by life change has been conducted by Thomas Holmes, M.D. at the University of Washington.[7] Dr. Holmes has clearly demonstrated that when stress-producing mothers-in-law visit or other disruptions occur, a person is far more prone to developing a bad cold or worse.[8] He studied patients who had colds and nasal infections, asking them when they came in for medical treatment to return upon recovery. As they returned, they were measured for blood flow, freedom of breathing, swelling and amount of secretion from the nose. Then he began to talk with them about the life events that had occurred before they became ill. After the conversation— about a mother-in-law, for example, or a new job—the measurements were repeated. It was discovered that the talk had renewed the cold symptoms.

Subsequent research has lead Holmes to conclude that there is a high correlation between life change and the onset of illness. His studies indicate any life change, desirable or undesirable, which requires coping or adaptive behavior can precipitate illness. These life change situations evolve from interpersonal and social transactions in the spheres of the family constellation, marriage, occupation, economics, residence, education, religion, recreation and health. Many of these events are part and parcel American values—achievement, success, materialism, self reliance. The studies confirm a correlation between life change and illness as innocuous as the common cold, and diseases as serious as tuberculosis. Holmes concludes, "If it takes too much effort to cope with the environment, we have less to spare for preventing disease." [7] The activity of coping can lower resistance to disease, particularly when one's copying techniques are faulty or when they lack relevance to the type of problems to be solved.

Holmes and an associate, Richard Rahe, M.D., have developed the Social Readjustment Rating Scale [9] which appears on page 43. They list 43 life change events in rank order of Life Change Units (LCU) representing the degree of adaptability required. For example, it implies that the death of one's spouse requires twice as much readjustment as getting married, four times as much as a change in living conditions and nearly 10 times as much as minor violations of the law.

The sum of the magnitudes of the life change items experienced in a given time determines the life change score for that interval. The higher the score the more likely the chance of a major health change.

To illustrate, Dr. Holmes suggests a hypothetical case.[7] Consider a singer who has finally hit the big time. What could be more gratifying? Concert tours, recording dates, parties, money and meeting famous people may well represent all of his dreams come true. But the way he lives his life will be radically changed. As the royalties begin to roll in (38) from his first hit record (28), he decides that his image needs updating, so he buys a new wardrobe and lets his hair grow long (24). He begins to work longer and longer hours at the recording studio for his new album (20) and then departs for a 3-month concert tour, staying in hotels and living out of a suitcase (25). He attends an endless string of parties and sees his old friends less and less (18). Concerts and parties keep him up most of the night, so he

Life Event	Mean Value
1. Death of spouse	100
2. Divorce	73
3. Marital separation	65
4. Jail term	63
5. Death of close family member	63
6. Personal injury or illness	53
7. Marriage	50
8. Fired at work	47
9. Marital reconciliation	45
10. Retirement	45
11. Change in health of family member	44
12. Pregnancy	40
13. Sex difficulties	39
14. Gain of new family member	39
15. Business readjustment	39
16. Change in financial state	38
17. Death of close friend	37
18. Change to different line of work	36
19. Change in number of arguments with spouse	35
20. Mortgage over $10,000	31
21. Foreclosure of mortgage or loan	30
22. Change in responsibilities at work	29
23. Son or daughter leaving home	29
24. Trouble with in-laws	29
25. Outstanding personal achievement	28
26. Wife begin or stop work	26
27. Begin or end school	26
28. Change in living conditions	25
29. Revision of personal habits	24
30. Trouble with boss	23
31. Change in work hours or conditions	20
32. Change in residence	20
33. Change in schools	20
34. Change in recreation	19
35. Change in church activities	19
36. Change in social activities	18
37. Mortgage or loan less than $10,000	17
38. Change in sleeping habits	16
39. Change in number of family get-togethers	15
40. Change in eating habits	15
41. Vacation	13
42. Christmas	12
43. Minor violations of the law	11

takes to sleeping in the day time instead (16). He has to stay on a strict diet to avoid getting paunchy and has to give up his beloved chocolate eclairs altogether (15). Whereas he used to play tennis twice a week and go sailing on weekends, now the most exercise he gets is tuning his guitar (19). His wife, initially delighted at the new excitement, finds that she is really not a part of his new life despite the fact that they have moved (20) into a new home. The couple argues more and more (35) about the time he spends away from home and their sexual relationship deteriorates (39).

The singer has accumulated 297 points in a short period of time. If his wife now begins seeing a psychiatrist (44) and files for a legal separation (65), he will find himself firmly in a position of high risk for experiencing some major change in health. In his particular profession, alcoholism or heavy drug use may be a likely possibility, but he might just as easily develop a bleeding ulcer or fall off the stage one night and break his leg.

Even if he tries to work things out with his wife by taking her on a vacation to Europe (13) and achieves a reconciliation with her (45), if he tries to go back to his former lifestyle it will only involve further changes in many of the spheres that he has already experienced.

What is your own risk? Take a moment and add up the score for all the items that apply to you in the last year. If you have recently experienced a major health change, chances are you had sufficient life-changes in the previous year to add up a score well in excess of 300. If your score is less than 150 over a one-year period, the risk of major health change in the next two years is about 33%. For a score of 150 to 299, the risk is about 50/50. If your score is well in excess of 300, you had better pay up your insurance. The risk of major health change is almost 90%. It must be pointed out that we all begin with a 10% chance of major health change.

This all sounds pretty grim, especially to those of us who continue to nourish the fantasy that some day soon everything is going to return to normal. One thing certain in life is that change is inevitable. The routine of our lives is constantly being revised. We must continually check out a flood of incoming stimuli, assign them priority, and assimilate them into our life-style. If we refuse to acknowledge their existence or are unable to cope with their frequency and intensity, our circuits may become overloaded with a massive life crisis and our systems are apt to break down.

Alvin Toffler has popularized this phenomenon under the general heading of *Future Shock* which he defines as "the distress, both physical and psychological, that arises from an overload of the human organism's physical adaptive system and its decision-making processes." [17]

Change is inevitable and often desirable. As we accomplish the developmental tasks in growing from childhood to adulthood, we change perspectives. New perspectives motivate different behaviors. Maturity brings a desire for change that represents improvement. Many of these changes are by choice. Other changes in our physical and social environment necessitating adjustments in our life-style are beyond our control. Some are undesirable and produce anxiety. That anxiety can cause us physical harm.

If change is inevitable, are we to assume that we are at the mercy of fate and other people? Not at all! Our response to change, not its frequency, should be the focal point of our attention. Our adaptability is the key to successful coping.

Dr. Holmes also suggests that we exert some control over change. We have a certain amount of personal control over whether and when to marry, go to college, move, or to have a family. We may have little control over whether to get divorced, change jobs, take out a loan, or retire. However, we may have a pretty good idea when these events may take place. With a degree of predictability we can order our lives by managing the change that is a vital part of living.

Changing, adapting and evolving help us to live our lives to our fullest capacity and enjoyment. However, too much change in too short a period of time takes its toll on the adaptive capabilities of the human body, lowers resistance and increases the risk of major changes in health. If we can learn to regulate the major changes that affect us, we may be able to defuse their consequences.

The Relationship of Emotion and Stress
to Malignancy

If emotion and the stress of life-changes can effect so many illnesses, what is their relationship to malignancy? As early as 1826, Sir Ashley Cooper claimed grief and anxiety to be among the most frequent causes of cancer. Psychological responses to cancer have long represented both interest and enigma to clinicians. More recently researchers have studied reactions of cancer patients to their illness. Reported findings indicate anxiety, fear and guilt predominate.

Other recent studies tie personality factors to the pathogenesis of cancer. In search for a personality profile of cancer patients, four characteristics have been reported: [16]

1. a tendency to hold resentment and a marked inability to forgive
2. a tendency toward self pity
3. inability to develop and maintain meaningful long-term relationships
4. poor self image

Of all the studies mentioned in this chapter, I believe this one to be the least credible. Any system devised to categorize human behavior leaves too wide a margin for error, and fails to allow for individual differences. In all the hundreds of patients with whom our staff has worked, we have rarely, if ever, observed all four of the above characteristics manifested in one person. It is, however, interesting to speculate that one who exhibits any of these negative behavior patterns may precipitate a physiological predisposition toward malignancy.

Several lengthy studies have documented loss of a significant love object six to eighteen months prior to diagnosis of cancer in many patients. Many believe this loss and an accompanying sense of rejection, helplessness and hopelessness to be a predisposing factor in the development of malignancy. The same researchers found a correlation between anxiety and rate of tumor growth in cancer patients. L. L. LeShan and R. E.

Worthington, Clinical Psychologists, found that patients with high anxiety experience rapid tumor growth, while those with low anxiety levels had slow growing tumors.

There are hundreds of articles in the medical literature which discuss the relationship of emotions and stress to malignancy. It is significant that all of them affirm a definite relationship between the two. There is little question as to whether emotions are a factor in cancer. The question is one of degree. Does the way we cope with life-change and stress affect our predisposition for contacting cancer? Can our coping style affect the physiological course of the disease after diagnosis? No study to date has given answers to these questions. The methodology has yet to be devised that will yield definitive proof of the degree of interaction between the mind and the body in relation to malignancy. There have been, however, some clinical experiences demonstrating the enhancement of medical treatment through the patient's positive mental perspective and skillful coping behavior.

One example is the placebo effect of aggressive but clinically ineffective medical treatment. The act of medical treatment in and of itself is encouraging to the patient. He has the satisfaction that something is being done to cope with his disease. Patients on a standard chemotherapy regimen often experience a high level of physical functioning, social adjustment and emotional stability even though the medication does not achieve the intended tumor control. When informed that the treatment has not controlled the malignancy, patients usually respond with a dramatic degeneration of mood and function. Patients who may have remained functional for months usually die soon after discovering that medical treatment has proven ineffective.

Some patients will opt for a course of treatment that holds little or no promise of disease control in order to buy time to complete unfinished business before they die. Even though the treatment may be totally ineffective, the act of doing something medical seems to give a needed sense of security. It is this phenomenon that keeps cancer quacks in business.

People who want to believe that a form of treatment is successful often experience temporary cessation of symptoms. Even though clinical tests confirm progression of the malignancy, patients who desperately want the treatment to succeed will feel better for a short time. Most peddlers of bogus cancer medications cannot produce clinical evidence of cancer regression or even confirm that their "cured" patients had a diagnosed cancer in the first place. One proponent of a bogus cancer drug reports only that his patients "feel better" after receiving his treatment. Few people realize that they have the right to demand evidence that a suggested medication has proven successful in other cases before consenting to receive it. Most qualified physicians will give patients statistical probabilities for success of a particular form of treatment before administering it. Most people will opt for the treatment even though the odds may be against success and they often feel better for a short time even if the treatment is ineffective.

Another example of the positive physiological effect of skillful coping behavior is the patient's ability to control specific symptoms such as pain and nausea. Pain from cancer is usually progressive due to rapid spread of malignancy and the degenerative process of the disease. For this reason, accomplishments in cognitive pain control have been less remarkable in cancer than in other physical disorders.

Pain clinics can train people with chronic lower back disorders to tolerate constant pain by changing their response to it. An individual's anticipation of pain often produces muscle tension and guarded movement which serve to intensify the pain. Learning to eliminate anticipatory muscle tension alleviates a large portion of the pain. By reprograming his cognitive behavior so he doesn't center his thinking and activity around pain, the patient achieves a more relaxed life-style. Even though similar approaches with pain from malignancy have not been especially successful, some cancer patients have achieved satisfactory pain control with little or no pain medication through cognitive conditioning such as relaxation therapy, self-hypnosis, and biofeedback.

Nausea induced by chemotherapy is a disconcerting side effect often controlled by a combination of antinausea drugs and cognitive conditioning. Vomiting subsequent to treatment is chemically induced. However, some patients experience an anticipatory anxiety response which induces nausea hours before treatment is administered. Pleasurable diversion during treatment, relaxation therapy and hypnotic suggestion have been successful in significantly reducing, or totally eliminating symptoms in many cases. Cognitive control of physiologic symptoms of cancer and its treatment is in its infancy. Recent intensification of interest in this area promises remarkable results in the future. Current experience exemplifies the positive control one can exercise over physiologic response.

Another example of mind over matter in cancer treatment can be observed in the approach of Carl Symonton, M.D.[16] Dr. Symonton is a radiation therapist who is attempting to demonstrate, through his clinical practice, the enhancement of physiologic response to medical treatment by cognitive conditioning. He hypothesizes that one's belief system has a positive or negative effect on one's response to treatment. He believes that if patients consider their cancer to be an uncontrollable destructive force outside themselves, and have a poor self-image or perceive medical treatment as bad, their response to therapy will be poor. If patients see themselves as victims, they will be. Conversely, Dr. Symonton believes that patients experience positive response to medical treatment when they see themselves in a position of control over the disease, believe the treatment will be effective and visualize their immune mechanisms as overcoming the malignant rebellion in the body.

Dr. Symonton, assisted by his wife, teaches his patients a technique they call relaxation and visualization. They describe it as a basic relaxation technique in which the patients are told to visualize their disease, their treatment, and their body's own immune mechanisms acting on the disease. The exercise is repeated three times a day during treatment. Patients are given a tape recording of the relaxation process and the book,

The Will to Live. They are invited to participate in group therapy sessions which reinforce the discipline of the mental imagery technique. Even though Dr. Symonton's research is too new to have produced statistically significant results, he feels confident that much will be learned regarding the impact on the length and quality of the patient's survival by influencing his attitude.

Finally, the individual's will to live and determination to function should never be underestimated. Dying patients often live long enough to accomplish specific goals they have set for themselves. I have seen many patients function under extremely adverse symptoms of pain and weakness—living long enough to resolve a conflict, be reunited with a relative, or accomplish a specific task—only to die within hours after accomplishing their goal.

Whether individual research efforts, such as Dr. Symonton's, will stand the test of clinical scrutiny remains to be seen. It is certain, however, that cancer patients can and do affect the length and quality of their survival through their coping behavior.

Conclusion

Is the body the servant of the mind? Solid clinical data indicates that at both the thinking and feeling levels our mental processes and emotions have a definite impact on the status of our health. Sometimes the impact is quite immediate. Sometimes it is the result of the cumulative effect of our adaptation to life-change events over a period of years.

Despite recent advancements in medical and psychosocial research, our understanding of the mind-body relationship is minimal. An exciting frontier in modern medicine is the exploration of the extent to which our mental and spiritual health can be employed to combat physical illness.

4

What about Faith Healing?

Given what is known of the impact of emotions and stress on physiological response, we are confronted by the question of faith healing. Does it occur? If so, how is it achieved? If it is successful with some, why not everyone? Has anyone ever been miraculously cured of cancer? How can we put this issue into perspective with reality?

Faith healing is nothing new. It has and continues to be a prevalent belief and practice in primitive societies. In our own culture it has deep roots in the quiet spiritual approach of Christian Science and its more demonstrative and emotionally charged counterparts—the evangelical and charismatic movements. William James in his classic, *Varieties of Religious Experience,* refers to all these as "mind cure methods." The emphasis in both approaches is on mind over matter in conjunction with a supernatural or divine power. On the one hand the *modus operandi* is to think only positive thoughts with the idea that a tranquil mind assures a healthy body. Christian Science does not recognize the existence of evil as reality, but only as "an error of the mortal mind." [1] According to this philosophy, if one does not acknowledge illness, one won't get sick.

The other extreme recognizes illness as a reality and calls on a supreme being or supernatural power to intervene on behalf of the patient. This is done by individual initiative, channeled through a faith healer, or through a social endeavor, such as the pilgrimages to Lourdes. In all faith healing experiences the common denominator for apparent success is the level of expectancy both of the patient and on the part of the healer.

The Role of Expectancy in Faith Healing

Primitive societies do not think in terms of the mind-body dualism of modern western culture.[15] They regard illness as a misfortune affecting the entire person, directly affecting relationships with the spirit world and with other members of the group. They do not distinguish sharply between mental and bodily illness or between natural or supernatural causes of illness. The power of the medicine man, witch doctor, or shaman is accepted as genuine and explained by the societies' world view. The shaman acquires his power through personal mystical experiences or through an elaborate training course analogous to medical training in our own culture. He is usually adept at distinguishing illnesses he can successfully treat from those that are beyond his powers, rejecting those patients with whom he is likely to fail. This enables him to maintain a reputation for success by arousing favorable expectations in the patient and the group, and undoubtedly enhances his healing power.

There are some striking similarities between the primitive shaman and the faith healer in western culture. Faith healers have usually received some formal training, education, and ordination from an established religious institution. It is believed that they have achieved or have been endowed with an additional dimension of divine power.

Faith healers are generally able to distinguish those cases with which they will be successful. I once attended the services of a nationally known faith healer. People with medically irreversible illnesses involving tissue regeneration or neurological repair were screened and placed in a location separate from the congregation. These were seen individually by the healer who had prayer with them, but were never presented in the open worship service.

The service itself was an interesting experience in suggestibility and mass hypnosis. A preliminary buildup of expectation preceded the healer's entrance. Emotionally stimulating gospel songs were sung. Specific rituals were performed to promote unity of thought and expectation. Worshipers were commanded to stand, raise their hands and declare, "I believe in miracles! I expect a miracle!" We were then instructed to turn and kneel at our seats and repeat prayers narrated by the leader.

After an hour of this activity, the healer appeared and exorted the congregation regarding the power and willingness of God to intervene in spiritual and physical illness. At the appointed time an invitation was extended for those who wished to be healed to come forward. Those who presented themselves had psychosomatic illnesses or symptoms which could be cognitively controlled.

This is not to say that healing did not take place or that such activity and belief is not without value. Pain is pain whether psychosomatic or organic in origin. The focal point is the role of expectancy in the success of faith healing.

Another case in point is an experimental demonstration in three severely ill and bedridden women.[4] One had chronic inflammation of the gall bladder with stones. The second had failed to recuperate from a major abdominal operation and was practically a skeleton. The third was dying from widespread cancer. The physician first permitted a prominent local faith healer to try to cure them by treating in absentia, without their knowledge. Nothing happened. Then the physician told the patients about the faith healer, built up their expectations over several days, and finally assured them that the faith healer would be treating them at a distance at a certain time the next day. This was at a time in which the physician was sure the healer would not be praying for them. However, at the suggested time the next day all three patients improved quickly and dramatically. The second was permanently cured. The other two were not, but showed striking temporary responses. The cancer patient who suffered severe anemia and fluid retention, promptly excreted all accumulated fluid, recovered from her anemia, and regained sufficient strength to go home and resume her household duties. She remained virtually symptom free until her death. The gall bladder patient lost her symptoms, went home and had no recurrence for several years. These three patients were helped by a belief that was false—that the faith healer was treating them from a distance —suggesting that what Leslie Weatherhead calls "expectant trust" in itself can be a powerful healing force.[18]

Popularity vs. Results

Healing cults are astonishingly popular. One physician found that 43% of his private patients had patronized a cult during the three months preceding their visits to him. Despite this popularity, overall statistics on the success of faith healing are not especially high. During the century it has existed, the famous healing shrine at Lourdes has had less than 100 cures pass the stringent requirements of the church to declare them miraculous. This figure may be conservative since many convincing cases lack the extensive documentary report required. But even several thousand cures of organic disease would represent only a small fraction of 1% of those making the pilgrimage. From forty to fifty thousand gather daily at the shrine. Visitors number in the millions annually. Of those, thirty thousand are patients.

The processes by which cures occur at Lourdes do not seem to differ in kind from those involved in normal healing. Careful reading of the reports reveals that healing is not instantaneous. However, consciousness of cure is often sudden and may be accompanied by immediate improvement of function. Actual tissue healing takes hours, days or weeks. People who have lost much weight require the usual time to regain it, as would be expected if healing occurred by the usual processes. Gaps of specialized tissues are not restored, but are filled by scar formation as in normal healing. No one has ever regrown an amputated limb at Lourdes.[4]

Inexplicable cures of serious organic disease occur in everyday medical practice. Two surgeons have assembled from the literature 176 cases of unquestionable cancer that regressed without adequate treatment. The authors stress that regression does not necessarily imply cure. However, about half of the cases were two years or more after cancer was diagnosed and about one eighth had been followed 10 years or more without recurrence. Had these remissions occurred after a visit to Lourdes or a faith healing service, they would be classified as miraculous. Since they cannot be explained by current medical theory, their cause remains open to question.

Another unanswered question in the issue of faith healing is why it seems to work for some and not others. Our clinical experience in five years at the Mountain States Tumor Institute yielded one patient who claimed that God had cured him. He refused further treatment. The patient had been diagnosed with an advanced incurable cancer. He returns annually for a checkup that reveals no clinical evidence of disease. Medically his case is described as a spontaneous remission. At least eight other patients made the same claim during this time period. They are all dead.

A dramatic case in point illustrating the opposite of spontaneous remission may be reported. A staff physician and I were summoned to confer with a patient who had not been referred by a physician, but who had walked in, asking for assistance. We were confronted by a middle-aged man holding a cloth to his face as he spoke. He explained that he did not desire medical treatment. He simply wanted a supply of surgical masks to cover a skin cancer on his face. The cancer had begun on his nose and spread, causing great pain and discomfort. He said that his cancer was a punishment for past sins. He had repented and now God was curing his cancer. He wanted the surgical masks to protect the lesion until the healing process was complete.

We suggested that physicians are men of God who employ his resources to hasten the healing process. He insisted that medical treatment was contrary to the tenets of his faith and that prayer and meditation was the only therapy he needed. When asked if his lesion had improved since his conversion, he reported cessation of pain and suggested that the physician examine the lesion and witness for himself the healing process. At this point, the man lowered the cloth, revealing an aggressive malignancy that had rendered him virtually faceless. Ironically, this was a cancer type that is very responsive to treatment. If treated early it could have been completely cured with an eight-week course of radiation therapy.

What Should a Patient Do?

In view of the data thus far discussed, how should the cancer patient regard the advisability or effectiveness of faith healing? On the one hand, western medical science views illness essentially as a malfunction of the body, correctable by medical and surgical interventions. On the other hand, there is the faith healer who promises to shortcut the laws of nature by direct divine intervention on behalf of the patient. Doubtless the truth lies somewhere between the two.

In the modern medical view of illness and treatment, physicians are highly skilled scientist/technicians. They diagnose a bodily disturbance in the human organism and correct it, much as a skilled mechanic would deal with a poorly running automobile. This approach to illness has enjoyed notable success and has elevated the physician to the exalted position of a modern shaman in the perception of most people. However, it is deficient in a crucial respect. It fails to acknowledge that psychological and bodily processes can profoundly affect each other. All illnesses have implications that may stimulate destructive emotional responses. Chronic illness with its constant misery, forced relinquishment of activities and roles which supported one's self-esteem and gave one's life significance, the threat of death—all may generate feelings of anxiety, hopelessness, and despair. When one's illness threatens the security of the patient's family, it may precipitate a progressive withdrawal on the part of both. Thus illness creates a vicious circle evoking emotions that aggravate it.

The insensitivity of scientific medicine to the potentially destructive effect of the emotions probably accounts for many of its failures, as well as impelling many patients to seek help from another source of healing. Faith healing, on the other hand, promises to arouse people's hope, bolster their self-esteem, stir them emotionally and strengthen their ties with a supportive group.

Equally outrageous is the physician who views patients only as disease entities, and faith healers who exploit the desperate hope of sick people with the fantasy that they can convince God to rewrite the laws of nature, just for them.

The cancer patient today has a better than even chance of achieving a healthy balance between scientific medicine and psychological support and guidance. With the mounting clinical evidence substantiating the impact of anxiety and stress on the quality and length of survival, psychosocial support will be an increasingly integral part of medical treatment planning.

All patients and their families must weigh the evidence and decide for themselves where they fit on the spectrum of effect of belief systems (faith) on physiological response. A good rule of thumb is to temper emotional stimulation with rational thinking based on known facts—cooperating with the laws of nature not trying to rewrite them.

Getting Perspective on Faith and Healing

The social alienation and threat of death from the modern leprosy often produce guilt in patients and generate intense interest in the meanings of life and faith. People who have been religious often become more so. Those who have not been religious often become more philosophical even if they do not affiliate with an institutional religious group. They have a basic need to find some coherence in human experience and a burning desire to "do things right," in order to preserve life and enhance its quality.

The next chapter will cover in detail specific techniques for coping with the cancer experience. In this section we will examine some dimensions of faith as a working philosophy for cancer patients and their families.

When Faith Is Recognition of Reality

One of the most frequent questions I am asked as a counselor to cancer patients is whether people with religious faith cope better. The answer is yes—provided their faith is active and alive. If one's faith is no more than a doctrinal system of statements that he believes should be true because someone said so, then his faith is not grounded in experience and will provide little support in times of crisis. Intellectual assent alone does not constitute a working philosophy.

Faith predicated on magical thinking is inadequate. Young children are prone to magical thinking. It is part of the mystery and wonder that makes childhood fun and children so enjoyable. But magical thinking can also become guilt-producing and destructive. A little girl who had gotten a new sled for Christmas prayed for snow. The very next day a snowstorm hit. With two feet of snow on the ground and more coming, the little girl became frightened at the destruction she thought she had brought on the world. That is amusing. But, when a child jumps from a second-story window because he thinks that he can fly like Superman, that is tragic.

When people carry their magical thinking into adulthood the results can also be tragic. The basis of childhood magical thinking is, "my thinking makes it happen." Do you remember how Jiminy Cricket sweetly sang, "A dream is a wish

your heart makes"? The song asserts that if you keep on believing strongly enough, your fondest dreams will come true.
And so Pinnocchio became a real boy. That is fine for Disney's
Fantasy Land, but it doesn't always work in real life. Parents
of a nine-year-old boy with terminal cancer were approached
by a church group who wanted to visit their home and pray
for the child. The parents agreed. The group came to the
home and prayed for God to heal the child. Upon leaving,
the spokesman told the mother, "If your faith is strong
enough, your son will be cured." Every day thereafter, a representative of the group phoned to ascertain whether the
symptoms were subsiding. The child died. The initial purpose
of the church group was to bring comfort and support. The
unrealistic expectations of their magical thinking brought, instead, increased anxiety and guilt.

If our faith is based on wishful thinking, we are set on a
painful collision course with reality. Cancer patients who
choose to deny the reality of the diagnosis or the severity of
the illness may, by inaction, hasten the death they are attempting to evade. A trip to the faith healer can also represent a
dangerous denial of reality. Time lost from proven forms of
medical care while one awaits divine intervention can be a futile and costly exercise in wishful thinking. The greatest trag-
edies in the field of cancer are the patients who waste away
the precious closing months of life in self-imposed isolation
awaiting a miracle that exists only in their own imagination.

Refusal to accept one's mortality is a negative use of the
denial mechanism, as well as a covert form of idolatry. Primitive people elevated to godly status anything more powerful
than themselves. A stone in the path that caused them to
stumble and fall was thought to have supernatural power.
They carried it back to their village as an object of worship.
Consequently, anything that threatened them with pain became an angry god which must be appeased. Cancer can
become a god to those who deny the reality of their mortality.
The emphasis of their lives is thrown out of perspective. All

their energy is directed toward the appeasement of the angry god, while the quality of their life disintegrates.

For example, a middle-aged man with terminal cancer perceived his illness as punishment for past sins. He had married a woman from another country and of a religious orientation diametrically opposite from that espoused by his family for generations. He had moved to her country and had converted to her faith. Through the years he became imprisoned by a sense of guilt. He became aware of the symptoms of the malignancy long before it was diagnosed. His guilt and fear prevented him from seeing a physician. The disease became widely disseminated and he could no longer deny its existence. When he realized the severity of his predicament, his cancer became an angry god to be appeased. He became obsessed with the desire that he and his family do everything "right." Failure to comply with his impossible expectations resulted in lengthy tirades. His compulsive abuse behavior sapped his energy and alienated his family.

The man sought the intercession of many clergymen. One pastor, who visited frequently, confided to a colleague that he felt divinely led to openly pray for a miraculous healing. His colleague warned that failure to achieve positive results would only increase the patient's sense of guilt with potentially disastrous results.

The attentive pastor continued to counsel his patient. He read comforting passages of Scripture which emphasized faith in the presence of adversity. He prayed silently for the patient's healing. After several months had lapsed, the pastor asked the patient if he felt any better as a result of their time together. "Yes," replied the patient, "I feel better inside."

Several days later, the man summoned his family to his bedside. He begged their pardon for imposing his outrageous expectations. He said, "I have tried to make you conform to my distorted sense of values for selfish reasons. Now I realize that I love you for what you are, not what I thought you should be. I am no longer afraid. I can die in peace."

Both the patient and his pastor learned that faith can restore a person to a sense of wholeness not necessarily meaning physical healing.

The charlatan faith healer flourishes on the mistaken notion that there is a dichotomy between science and faith. For many, faith is a dark reservoir in which to dump anything unexplainable. Georgia Harkness affirms "much trouble would be saved by getting it clearly in mind at the outset that religious ideas, like any other ideas, can be true only when they are tied to reality and tested by the whole of life." [6]

The Bible defines faith as "assurance of things hoped for, a conviction of things not seen." The passage then describes how the saints of old tested their faith. All the great scientific discoveries are an outgrowth of faith tested by reality. Each discovery began with an assurance of hope and a conviction that something not yet clearly understood existed and could be constructively used. Our homes are lighted with incandescent bulbs because Edison had a conviction of things unseen. Our children are free from the threat of polio because Jonas Salk had an assurance of something hoped for. Penicillin was discovered because Alexander Flemming was convinced that there was more to be seen in bread mold than its greenish color. Thousands of cancer patients are now being cured because the Curies, through the assurance of hope and conviction, were able to isolate and harness an unseen energy in a substance called radium.

What works for the scientist should work for the religious. Leslie Weatherhead said it best: "Faith is not a leap in the dark, as the schoolboy said, 'believing what you know to be untrue,' or treading a road that is contrary to reason and superstitiously running in another direction. It is taking the road of evidence as far as it will go and then, with the energy provided by meditating on the character of God as Christ revealed him, making a leap of faith, only to land finally in a conviction as strong as proof can supply." [18]

Essential to the quality of life for the cancer patient is a working philosophy based on the recognition and acceptance of reality.

When Faith Is Acceptance of Personal Responsibility

Elizabeth Kübler-Ross has described the bargaining mechanism as one in which patients attempt to buy a postponement of death.[12] She tells of patients bargaining with God or a physician by promising to devote the rest of their lives to the church or donating their bodies to science. This bargaining always places the burden of responsibility on someone other than the patient. We might define it as an unrealistic attempt to manipulate persons or circumstances in an effort to evade the inevitable.

When this mechanism is used, the burden of responsibility is always placed on someone else. The patient is overwhelmed with the prospect of an incurable disease and feels powerless to effect a change in this condition. Such patients focus on a source of power outside themselves and attempt to buy it. The danger is twofold. On the one hand is the futility of unrealistic expectations. On the other hand, this approach reinforces dependency and intensifies helplessness. Moreover, it is a cop-out. Patients who accept their portion of responsibility in their care plan exert control over their environment and their disease. They enhance their response to medical therapy and increase their level of functioning. Dr. Symonton reports that the most successful patients in his program are those who are willing to accept responsibility for the impact of their belief system on their physiological response.

I recall as a child being taught in Sunday school that God, through Christ, has done for us what we cannot do for ourselves. I have since observed many practicing Christians asking God to do for them what they *won't* do for themselves. My father was a practical Methodist parson. One of his most memorable sermons was an exposition of the text: ''The effectual fervent prayer of a righteous man availeth much.'' Dad used a modern translation, ''A good man can do a great deal with prayer—when he tries.'' In the cancer center I have seen many clinical demonstrations of the truth of which he spoke—courageous patients who never let their limitations blind them to their strength; whose faith is a working philosophy—not a cop-out from personal responsibility.

When Faith Is Trust, Not Neurotic Dependency

A working philosophy that can provide practical support is one that exercises trust rather than neurotic dependency.

Neurotic dependency is the manifestation of a basic insecurity often reinforced by an unwillingness to cultivate coping skills commensurate with one's ability. Adverse circumstances serve to increase feelings of helplessness, hopelessness, and inadequacy. Often people around a patient reinforce dependency so that the individual acquiesces, adopting it as a way of life. Until the patients take the risk of reliance, they will never learn what latent strength they possess.

Trust involves relaxed reliance and confident commitment as opposed to the anxious grasping and defensive possessiveness of neurotic dependency. In human relationships this means that when we have a clear understanding of our own capabilities and limitations we are free to trust a part of ourself and our responsibilities to another. Having recognized reality and accepted personal responsibility, we are free to receive graciously as well as to give freely. In receiving we do not feel put down, nor do we give in order to achieve a feeling of superiority.

When I was a small boy, I fell overboard while playing on the docks. I became hysterical, clutching the side of a rowboat, thrashing wildly in the water and screaming frantically for someone to help me. My father stood calmly on the dock and quietly suggested that I stand up. "I can't," I screamed, "I'll drown, and you don't even care!" In a stern voice my father commanded, "Son, stop blubbering and stand on your own two feet." I stopped screaming and did as he suggested, only to discover that I was in water barely up to my waist. My father taught me the meaning of trust.

Cancer patients who know their capabilities and accept personal responsibility are able to maintain their optimum level of physical function within the constraints of the illness. By freely accepting assistance only when needed, they keep expectations of support from others in a realistic perspective. By placing no inordinate expectations on others, they enhance their interpersonal relationships which, in turn, reinforce their own positive self-image. Cancer patients who exercise trust can significantly increase the quality of their lives.

Conclusion

Solid clinical data indicate that psychological processes have a definite impact on physiological response. This impact can be either negative or positive in terms of illness and health. The role of expectation seems to be of paramount significance in both scientific medicine and so-called faith healing. While I would not dispute the positive effect of faith on the healing process, it is recommended that the emotional stimulation of religious feelings be tempered with reality-oriented decision-making. Searching for the quick miraculous cure can represent failure to accept reality, evasion of personal responsibility, and a basic insecurity that undermines trust. When we confuse our egocentric expectations with faith in God, we run the risk of separating ourselves from his love if they are not in harmony with his design.

5

Coping with Cancer: Reorientation

All technical wonders of modern medical science notwithstanding, our broadest sympathies and deepest anxieties are stimulated when we hear about someone we know having cancer. When we are honest with ourselves most of us will admit that being around cancer patients is threatening to us. If the life situation of these patients is at all comparable to our own, we personally identify with them. We experience a crushing sense of inadequacy when we mentally put ourselves in their place. Our sense of inadequacy produces anxiety. Our anxiety causes us to put a safe distance between ourselves and the source of discomfort. Our conversations with them become guarded, relationships superficial. Perhaps a large measure of our anxiety stems from not knowing how they may respond to what we say. Personal contacts become less frequent as we find comfort in the out-of-sight, out-of-mind syndrome.

But what if the crisis did not always happen to the other person? What if one day I found myself in a physician's office and heard the words: "I am sorry to be the bearer of bad news, but . . ." I say to myself, "Can this really be happening to me? Surely there is some terrible mistake." Then comes the chilling realization that those strange sensations I have been feeling were symptoms of malignancy growing and spreading in my body. Is there any hope? Can something be done? Will it be painful? Will I suffer? What shall I tell my wife? She is still young. Surely she will find someone else when I am gone. I am not sure I like that idea either. How much time do I have? Will I see my children grow up? My God! When I think of all I had planned for the future I realize how much of myself and my time I have wasted on trivia.

If you are a patient or relative of a patient, you know the disorienting and disintegrating effect of a cancer diagnosis. It becomes difficult to focus thinking or coordinate function. Anxiety is an early warning system that trouble is crouching at the door.

Converting Anxiety to Fear

The initial anxiety experienced upon diagnosis of cancer is disorienting largely because it is nondescript and out of focus. Unfocused anxiety or suspicion is disorienting and destructive because it presents the patient with an unknown adversary. It is essential for the patient and family to express their feelings, to get them outside in the light of day where they can be seen clearly. As anxieties are verbalized they begin to take the shape of specific fears. Nondescript anxieties converted into focused fears give the adversary dimensions that can be confronted. Focused fear is the first step in reorientation.

Facing Fear

Fear itself can paralyze positive thought and action. Facing fear and using it to our advantage is essential to successful coping with the adversary whether it is cancer, an angry boss, or the bully across the street. Studies at the Mountain States Tumor Institute in comparative anxiety levels of patients indicate that patients who are unable to say, "I have cancer," have problems adjusting to the cancer experience. Being able to verbalize fears helps in confronting and overcoming them.

The son of one patient assisted her with this task. He had come to visit his mother in the hospital after her surgery for breast cancer and the conversation went something like this:

SON: "How extensive was your surgery, Mother?"

MOTHER: "The surgeon removed my breast."

SON: "Why?"

MOTHER: "You know, a cyst."

SON: "Just a cyst, Mother?"

MOTHER: "Well, you know . . . a tumor."

SON: "What kind of tumor, Mother?"

MOTHER: "Well, you know, a mass."

SON: "Come now, Mother, was the tumor benign or malignant?"

MOTHER: "Well, I guess . . . it was malignant."

SON: "Come on Mother, say it. Say the words, I have cancer."

MOTHER: "I have cancer."

SON: "There now, you are not any different for having said the word, are you? You are not any less a person for having cancer. We all still love you just as much. Don't be afraid to talk about it. The only way to beat it is to face it."

This particular person had been consumed by her fear of cancer. She went into surgery thinking that even if she lived through the operation her life span would be extremely limited. She had many other fears to face. She perceived the cobalt machine as some sort of voodoo instrument. However, she continued with treatment in spite of her fears. She adjusted well to the loss of her breast and overcame her fear of cobalt, and cancer in general. She lived five years without any clinical evidence of disease. At the end of that time the cancer returned to her spine creating severe pain which temporarily confined her to bed. She responded well to treatment and is currently on maintenance chemotherapy. While her physical activity is limited, she is ambulatory, happy, and a well adjusted person. Her motto, "Cancer isn't half as bad the second time around."

Living With Uncertainty

Chronic Versus Acute Illness

The anxiety of living with uncertainty is another formidable adversary of the person with cancer. With acute illnesses we take our treatment, go through a brief period of convalescence, and then go on our way never again giving the illness a second thought. Even those sick people belonging to the fellowship of sufferers, who enjoy comparing operations and showing scars, have the satisfaction of knowing that illness is behind them. The satisfaction of knowing that illness has been overcome makes the bragging all the better. In contrast, people who have cancer must adjust to the probability that they will never be cured. Even when there is no clinical evidence of the disease the threat of its return is always present. One patient said:

> When I am feeling good I find myself wanting to forget that I ever had it. Then I go to the mirror and tell myself that I have cancer, so that when it returns the shock will not be too great. With all they know about this disease there is no way the medics can prevent its return. Let's face it, having cancer is a floating crap game.

Checking the Options

The first step in learning to live with uncertainty is developing the ability to check available options and the freedom to take calculated risks. This means one must be able to distinguish between realistic hope and rainbow chasing. If the person with incurable cancer nourishes false hope for cure the foundation for all future action is built on very shaky ground. Like the biblical parable, the house that is built on sand simply cannot withstand the shock of the storm.

In treating cancer, if cure is not possible, long term control is the next option. If neither is a realistic goal, relief of symptoms and alleviation of pain becomes the hope on which future plans are based. The patient and his family need to know which of these options are open to them. If cure is even a remote possibility, any of us would pursue it with vigor. But what of the costs: financial, physical, emotional, and social? What medical procedures will be necessary? Will treatment alter appearance or body function? Will it be painful? What adjustments will be necessary in life-style? Will those adjustments be temporary or permanent? All these questions should be asked. Answers should be given by the physician, and clearly understood by the patient and family.[14]

Setting Expectations

The expectations of the patient and his family regarding response to treatment and future outcome should correlate with those of the health care team. Most of us have difficulty in assimilating medical information especially under stress of a cancer diagnosis. It usually takes several explanations before medical options are clearly understood. In institutions where a team approach is used, other members of the staff, such as the nurse, social worker, and chaplain, can be of great assistance in nonmedical aspects of the disease. They can also assist patients and families to focus on specific medical questions to present to the physician.

Having been informed of the diagnosis, prognosis, and treatment plan, the most prevalent questions posed by patients are, "Is it worth it all? If I am going to die anyway, why not spare us all the pain and cost and let nature take its course?" Faced with difficult decisions regarding health and life many people are tempted to relinquish responsibility and control, and to resign from the human race. Even though the stakes of the game are high it is usually worth the calculated risk involved. Medical procedures are not usually recommended unless there is realistic hope for response.

Carl Jung pointed out that the meaning of life comes not in solutions to problems, but in search of solutions. In the final analysis, learning to live with uncertainty, by checking viable options and taking calculated risks, is the most sensible way of facing the reality of a world that offers few guarantees.

One Day at a Time

When goals for living within constraints of the disease have been established and a course of action has been chosen, the patient and his family then need to take life one day at a time. Having received the most expert advice available together with our own best thoughts and actions, it is time for us to rest secure in our decision and give life the best shot we have.

Once the program has been launched in cancer treatment, "wait and see" is the name of the game. It takes weeks, even months, before response to some forms of treatment can be determined. During that time there are many tests and much waiting and wondering. But which of us can add one minute to the span of our lives by being anxious. Don't worry about tomorrow. Tomorrow will take care of itself. Today's concerns are sufficient for today. An ancient prayer is apropos: "God grant me the serenity to accept those things I cannot change, the courage to change the things I can, and the wisdom to know the difference."

Learning to live with uncertainty teaches us something about quality versus quantity of life by giving it our best shot one day at a time. This experience has led one man to begin a mutual support movement among cancer patients called "Make Today Count." [11]

Dimensions of Adaptability

The sweeping changes in life-style and physical function experienced by many patients with cancer precipitates a psychological and social crisis. Adaptive skills are required of both patient and family in order to regain equilibrium. People who have learned to cope effectively with past crises usually do quite well. Others must develop new skills in order to facilitate rehabilitation. Research at Mountain States Tumor Institute has identified various dimensions of adaptability. People who have developed a high degree of adaptability in each area usually adjust well on their journey with cancer. Those who have not developed these coping skills during past crises could benefit from professional help to facilitate rehabilitation.

1. *Self-disclosure* — Patients who can freely express their thoughts and feelings regarding the illness will adapt more easily than those who cannot.

2. *Responsiveness to thoughts and feelings of others* — Patients and families who are responsive to the thoughts and feelings of each other will cope better than those who talk but do not listen.

3. *Role flexibility*—Patients and family members who can accept temporary or permanent role changes will cope better. For example, the breadwinner who can easily accept the role of patient during the acute phase of illness, and later, return to work, demonstrates a high degree of adaptability. The working wife who can accept the additional temporary role of nurse with equanimity will facilitate her husband's rehabilitation.

4. *Quality of relationship*—The patient and family who share feelings and responsibilities will adapt better than those who do not.

5. *Degree of participation*—Patients whose family members participate in the planning and providing of care will re-

spond better to treatment than those whose families relinquish responsibility.

6. *Satisfaction with medical care*—Patients who have been satisfied with previous medical care and demonstrate confidence in their physician will respond better to treatment.

7. *Participation in decision-making*—Patients who are included in the medical and nonmedical decision-making will be more easily rehabilitated than patients who are excluded by the medical treatment team and/or family.

8. *Quality of support*—Patients whose family members provide appropriate physical and emotional support will respond better than those whose families are unable to provide such support.

9. *Positive reinforcement versus aversive control* — Patients and families who rely on positive reinforcement in their interpersonal relationships will adjust to the cancer experience. Those who rely on aversive control will probably experience disintegration of relationships. This dimension will be discussed in greater detail later in the chapter.

Coping with Depression

Depression is usually the result of feelings of helplessness. At this point a distinction should be drawn between temporary feelings of sadness and pathologic depression. Everyone experiences temporary feelings of sadness after a bad day, or following a set of circumstances that represent a crisis. Clinical depression is defined as a period of time when one's level of physical function and interpersonal transactions are disrupted. This may be characterized by difficulty in eating and sleeping, persistently cold hands or feet, inability to accomplish routine tasks and an uncommunicative or withdrawn attitude. If these symptoms persist for an extended period of time—weeks or months—the depression may be termed pathological and professional help is required.

When people with cancer become depressed it is usually because they are responding appropriately to very disturbing circumstances. When one has been given reasonable assurance of cure, a strong depression reaction is inappropriate. However, those faced with far advanced disease with no guarantees of cure or response to treatment have good reason to be depressed. When depression occurs under these circumstances it is usually a sign that the patients are adjusting to their situation through a natural process of mourning.

It is disconcerting for those close to the patient to see their loved one grieving and downcast. Usually, the first reaction is to want to do or say something to "snap them out of it." It is important for those around the patient to understand that no one can get another person out of a depression. No one can be totally responsible for another's thoughts and actions. When a mood of depression exists we can only help by providing a supportive environment conducive to positive response. There are several guidelines for interaction that might be helpful.

First, *thou shalt not refuse someone the temporary luxury of self pity when there are reasons for feeling depressed.* Sorrow expressed by one we love may be threatening. Failure to grant permission for expression of honest feelings stimulates a sense of rejection and erodes the integrity of the relationship. This is not to encourage maudlin sentimentality or suggest group hysteria. It is simply to recommend letting the patient know that it is OK to have feelings of depression and that those feelings are not only understood, but shared.

Sitting quietly while a depressed person cries, and giving a reassuring touch of the hand is often far more supportive than any words we may speak. Sometimes it is appropriate for family members to cry together. Crying is an expression of caring that cannot be demonstrated any other way. That form of emotional release is an appropriate way of working through depression. Some do not like to "let down" in front of the patient. They may feel that it signifies they are beginning to crumble under the stress, or that they are not strong enough to bear up with courage. Crying acknowledges the reality of unpleasant circumstances. Some have the mistaken feeling that as long as the adversary is not openly acknowledged everything will be all right. When coping with the cancer crisis that behavior may be classified as rainbow chasing.

Some men do not like to cry because they feel it is effeminate and shows lack of courage. Elizabeth Kübler-Ross has correctly stated, "It takes a strong man to cry." [12]

A second guideline for supporting the depressed patient is: *Thou shalt not patronize with worn-out cliches, but focus on realistic hope.* Statements of encouragement that are not based on realistic hope are more destructive than saying nothing at all. Give the patient an opportunity to work through depression by expressing his feelings. Then focus on what can be realistically expected given the circumstances.

A third guideline is: *Thou shalt be supportive, not controlling.* The basic responsibility for working through depression rests with the patients. In the final analysis, they are the ones who have control over their feelings. When they choose to exert that control their mood will change. Those around them should not reinforce their depression by assuming control. The use of patronizing clichés are a put-down. Attempts to "do something" to get them out of the dumps serves only to reinforce their feelings that they are out of control of the situation. Giving the patients control of their lives by including them in the treatment process and family decision-making will enhance the quality of life for them and reduce the possibility of their feeling helpless.

For the patients, maintaining control should not mean lying in bed shouting out orders. It involves instead exerting control over their own thoughts and feelings, in order to maintain a high level of physical and mental function. Feeling sad about adverse circumstances is natural. Dwelling on sadness and self-pity is debilitating. It solidifies one's self-image into helplessness. The challenge to exert self-control and positive action is essential.

Open Communication

No problem can be confronted and dealt with rationally without open communication. This is especially true in the cancer experience. Free expression of thought helps us keep in touch with our feelings and provides a therapeutic emotional catharsis in times of stress and crisis. There may be feelings of anger, frustration, doubt, fear, helplessness, suspicion, and despair. These initial feelings will probably be temporary as well as somewhat disproportionate to the situation. Free expression is necessary for the patients to get their feelings out where they can deal with them, to hear themselves say what they feel in order to gain perspective and an element of control.

Equal in importance to free expression and self-determination is the ability to listen. Current research at MSTI indicates that patients whose families fail to consider their thoughts and feelings and do not include them in decision making may not respond fully to medical treatment. Also, these patients must be at risk in terms of psychological and social adaptability. Do they feel differently about themselves now that they have cancer? Do they feel information is being withheld from them by the medical staff or family? Do they perceive their friends relating differently to them now that they have cancer? What are their expectations of treatment, of the future, and of the family? Does the family perceive the patient's role as changing? In what role does the patient see other family members? Straight answers to these and many other questions are necessary to prevent breakdown in communication and preserve the integrity of relationships.

Essential to open communication is the ability to pin-point feelings and check inferences regarding the thoughts of others. Voice intonation, facial expression or specific behaviors all lead to conclusions about each other's thoughts. However, a single frown can indicate any one of a number of reactions: anger, pain, frustration, or a minor gastrointestinal disturbance portending imminent social embarrassment. Misinterpretation of the frown may lead to a misunderstanding that jeopardizes the relationship.

Social Reinforcement

Social Learning

The social dimension of coping with the cancer crisis is critical. Individuals can exert control over their own thoughts and feelings. However, one cannot do it alone. Positive thinking and behavior must be reinforced by the patient's family or support group.

Effective interdependence is the most productive way patients and their families can interact with one another. The principles of social reinforcement learning have much to teach us in this regard.

The essence of this theory asserts that we learn by social response which behaviors are socially acceptable and which are inappropriate. The way we feel about ourselves and the way we interact with others are largely socially learned. The learning process for each individual begins with parents and continues with authority figures and peers. Acceptable and appropriate behavior is reinforced with rewards. Unacceptable or inappropriate behavior is either punished or ignored.

Learning can take place through cognitive conditioning. The teacher explains, the pupil feeds back the explanation orally or in writing. This is a social process in which learning is rewarded by a high score, while failure is punished by a low score.

Learning also occurs through a process of modeling and imitation. If a boy imitates the behavior of his chosen hero and grows up to be pastor of the church or president of the company everybody is happy. If, on the other hand, he follows a less socially acceptable model and joins a terrorist group there may be much grieving.

The Pain Behavior Clinic at the University of Washington is an outstanding example of how social learning principles can be applied in health care. Under the direction of Dr. William Fordyce this clinic serves people with chronic back pain that can never be completely corrected by medical treatment. Through a process of social learning the patient's response to pain is altered even though the physiologic cause of the pain is not changed.

When people think about how badly they hurt it serves to accentuate pain. When they talk about it to others the sympathetic responses they receive reinforce pain behavior. The patient's mode of walking, facial expression, physical function, and social interactions all revolve around pain. They think, feel, and act pain. At the Pain Behavior Clinic, discussion of pain is avoided. Complaints about pain are ignored. Patients receive positive reinforcement for behaving as though they were pain free and governing physical activity to minimize pain. At the end of five weeks of therapy, many patients exhibit a dramatic change in mood, movement, and affect. They return to their home environment making periodic visits to the clinic for refreshers of reinforcement behavior learning.

Positive Reinforcement Versus Aversive Control

Cancer patients are introduced to a foreign world of medical specialties that overwhelm them with confusing terminology and painful procedures. The medical experts hold the key to life and death. The patients are tempted to relinquish control of their lives in exchange for a piece of the future. Many of the rewarding experiences—reinforcers—they were once able to enjoy fade into the oblivion of yesterday. These experiences are gone, but not forgotten. It all happens so fast there isn't time to think. The patients have to act fast, get on the treatment program, and not let cancer take over. They may begin to experience a deeper fear than they have ever known. The specter of death hovers with prominent finality. The feeling of encroaching helplessness induces the fear of abandonment.

It is at this point that sensitive appropriate social reinforcement is imperative to quality of life. Research at MSTI indicates that patients adapt better when families rely on positive reinforcement rather than aversive control in interpersonal relationships.

Aversive control is the stubborn silent refusal of a husband to say tender and affectionate phrases he knows his wife longs to hear. It is the inordinate contingencies a woman may place on the bestowal of her favors to her husband. Aversive control is the verbal slur calculated to put someone down. It is the stony silence with which a preoccupied parent turns a deaf ear to a child's simple request.

Positive reinforcement is a reassuring touch of the hand in anxious or despairing moments. It is unsolicited verbal praise. Positive reinforcement is refraining from verbal abuse while your children are learning from a mistake. It is listening to them when they share a serious problem or a joke that tickles their funny bone, but leaves you cold.

When cancer patients have lost rewarding social contacts, family and friends can be of valuable assistance. For example, during the period of recovery from a surgical procedure walking from the bed to the bathroom may be the equivalent of a week's work. Encouragement to go it alone with firm praise for success is comparable to a raise in pay. Ignoring unnecessary bids for sympathy and assistance is an appropriate way of refusing to give reinforcement for inappropriate behavior.

At this point it is appropriate to emphasize again the benefit of positive reinforcement by giving the patient an element of control in the treatment process. This can be illustrated by the use of relaxation therapy to control the pre-treatment anxiety response of vomiting. Nausea and vomiting subsequent to treatment is a prevalent side effect with some chemotherapeutic drugs. This stimulates such stress in some patients that their anticipatory anxiety precipitates the post-treatment symptoms long before the treatment is administered.

Use of relaxation therapy has produced some remarkable results in alleviating this pre-treatment anxiety response. With this form of intervention patients are taught the life skill of voluntary stress control. This is accomplished by means of an audio tape cassette to which the patient listens for an hour each day for about one week. Through systematic tensing and relaxing body and facial muscles the patient is made aware of the sensations of deep relaxation. When the entire body is totally relaxed the patients are instructed to repeat the word "calm" each time they exhale and to associate the word with the body sensation of deep relaxation and a sense of peace and well being. After a week of practice the patients have mastered the skill of deep relaxation by simply lying prone and mentally repeating the word "calm" each time they exhale.

One patient had experienced a severe pre-treatment anxiety response which induced nausea and vomiting several hours before each treatment. Prior to her relaxation therapy she would experience violent symptoms the moment she awoke on the day of treatment. She came to the clinic tense and drawn, clutching her husband's arm. After mastering the skill of voluntary stress control, the change was dramatic. She awoke refreshed and happy on the day of treatment, came to the clinic and went to sleep during the treatment. Her post-treatment symptoms were also considerably less severe.

Through this therapeutic method the patient was taught to take control of her own responses. Her successful self-control was a form of positive reinforcement to her self esteem. With the disappearance of her pre-treatment anxiety her husband's anxiety was relieved and their relationship enhanced.

The Danger of Denial

Studies have indicated that cancer patients who are well integrated mentally and emotionally stable live longer. The same studies indicate that those who choose to deny intensely the threat of cancer also live longer. A superficial denial mechanism may be an appropriate form of determination that keeps the patient functional. However, perpetual use of a deep seated denial mechanism can be a threat to the patient's physical wellbeing and family relationships. Well-integrated people are in touch with their own feelings, sensitive to others and open in their communication. They set realistic goals and accomplish them. When they die, both they and their survivors have the satisfaction of personal fulfillment. Little has been left unsaid or undone.

In contrast, people who choose to ignore reality tend to become withdrawn and self-centered. As they lose more control over their physical condition they become more demanding. They set unrealistic expectations for themselves and others. The pursuit of their impossible dream becomes the all consuming goal of life. They no longer hear what others say to them. They turn off any words that do not reinforce their fantasy and sever communication with those who will not play their game. When the crushing reality that they have lost control over the disease finally dawns, they often despair and die an empty and lonely death leaving their survivors emotionally depleted.

Impairment Need Not Mean Disability

Those confronting the cancer crisis are faced with some stark realities through which they can learn the difference between quality and quantity of life; between realistic hope and chasing rainbows. They can learn how to adapt in such a way that even a permanent physical impairment need not become a disability. Mastery of these lessons will assure them a solid personal victory regardless of the length of life. On the other hand, if they are not rational, adaptive, and decisive they may make a profession of this illness, and their lives will be wasted.

The most angry patient I ever saw was a man who had made a profession of his illness. He had never learned to develop durable human relationships based on trust and mutual respect. He had never mastered even basic social skills with his family and friends. Instead, he relied on coersion and aversive control in his personal interactions. His cancer diagnosis stimulated sympathetic support from those he had previously alienated. Now he enjoyed attention he had not experienced in years. After treatment his cancer went into remission. When his physician announced that there was no clinical evidence of disease, his passport to automatic sympathy disappeared. His reaction was intense anger toward the physician who had taken away the crutch from his sick personality.

Making a profession of illness is nothing new in human history. The Bible tells the story of a man who had been paralytic for many years. He spent all of his time by the pool of Bethzatha. According to the legend of the day, when the surface was rippled by the flutter of an angel's wings, the first person to enter the pool would be healed. Somehow, someone else always got into the pool before he could. He finally came to expect others to beat him to it. Apparently those around him also expected him to continue in the sick role so he made a profession of his illness. He had allowed his impairment to become a permanent disability. No one had ever challenged him to anything more than lying on a mat beside the pool nurturing broken dreams. He developed a poor self image. What that man needed was someone to challenge him to assert himself and make the best with what he had.

One day a stranger came by. He was called Jesus of Nazareth. He had an innate ability to confront people with the truth about themselves in a way that reinforced self-confidence rather than putting them down. He asked the man, "Do you want to be healed?" The sick man did not answer the question directly. He just muttered some excuses for not getting into the pool. Jesus challenged the paralytic to assert himself; to exert some control over his life rather than surrendering his responsibility to the chance that something miraculous might someday occur. All that in the simple imperative, "Pick up your bed and walk." The man tried it and succeeded!

One of the most effective members of the staff at our cancer center in Boise is a medical technologist. Judy has a severe physical impairment. Paraplegic with limited use of her hands, she is confined to a wheelchair. I don't know the origin of Judy's physical problems. Neither do the other staff members, including those who help her to the lady's room for nature breaks. It never occurs to us to ask her. She never talks about it, why should we? Even though Judy hasn't enough strength in her arms to propel her wheelchair, she draws blood from her patients with painless tenderness and the superlative skill of a highly trained surgeon. She is empathetic, not sympathetic. With quiet dignity she personifies strength and courage to people who might otherwise be inclined to feel sorry for themselves.

Because she lives with a physical impairment, cancer patients often identify with her and develop a reciprocal relationship none of the rest of us could ever achieve. Her positive self-image is catching. Once a dying patient who had been a pilot had come into the clinic several days in succession in deep depression. He was a big man physically and had represented a tower of strength to patients and staff alike. It was threatening to everyone to see him depressed and dying. He had loved life and filled every minute with sixty seconds worth of distance run. Now he was down and needed someone to talk with, but no one seemed to know what to say. It is difficult to say goodbye to someone you respect and don't want to see die.

He came into the clinic that day the picture of dejection, slumped into the chair at the lab, and stretched out his arm for the blood test with the automatic detachment of a robot. Judy took his hand gently and began her work. "You look depressed," she said. With a deep lingering sigh he asserted, "I think that I am on my last flight." Their eyes met and after a long moment Judy said, "Well, if you have to go, fly first class!" A big smile broke the clouds of depression as he stood tall and walked erect from the lab. The man never returned to the clinic. He flew first class the next day.

By learning the difference between realistic hope and chasing rainbows Judy has developed a positive self-image and has not allowed impairment to become a disability. She could have denied reality and nurtured the false hope that some day someone would find a miracle cure for her condition. She may have dreamed of someday becoming an Olympic athlete, or, in Cinderella fashion, dancing into the night with her Prince Charming. Instead, she confronted reality and made the best of what she had. She has compensated with mental ability for all that she lacks in physical strength. She holds a baccalaureate degree in Biology and Medical Technology. In addition to working directly with patients, she manages the lab, supervises two other medical technologists and conducts significant research projects of her own design. Some results of her research have been published in professional journals. She goes to football games and likes boys.

It all sounds easier than it really is. Simple functions taken for granted by most people are difficult procedures for Judy— combing her hair, taking a shower, getting dressed in the morning, cutting her meat. She lives with a constant fear of failure or that a sudden lack of muscular control will cause her to inflict pain on one of her patients. Instead of giving in to her fears and quitting she uses her fears to increase her human sensitivity. There are many things that she can't do for herself. She must rely on help from others. Being independent and still graciously accepting help from others for basic functions is a difficult lesson to learn, both for the individual and for those around him. Judy's family and close associates at work are always available, but never patronizing.

Through Judy's experience we have all learned something of the value of effective interdependence.

Conclusion

Patients who are willing to confront the realities of their illness and exert some control in the decision-making process of treatment planning, home life, and work activity will retain their positive feelings of self worth. Giving the patients control places responsibility equally on them, the family, and the health care team. The patients must be willing to deal with their situation. The family must not give in to the desires to "protect" the patient by withholding information. The physician and other members of the health care team must not assume a role of omniscience, and must be willing to negotiate with the patient in treatment planning. It is not our purpose, at this point, to enter a lengthy discussion of patient's rights but simply to point out that any measure taken to give the patients reasonable control is paramount in enhancing the quality of their survival.

Families that are free to permit patients to ventilate their honest hopes and fears, and share their own, promote stability and emotional security. If they are strong enough to ignore, rather than punish inappropriate behavior, giving positive reinforcement to honest effort, they become agents of functional maintenance for the patient. Not in spite of, but because of the cancer experience, they will know the ultimate sense of fulfillment in becoming members one of another.

6

Children
and Cancer

Suffering innocence always evokes universal sympathy. The thought of a child victimized by cancer brings to the surface our strongest feelings of indignant anguish. Why should an innocent child with a whole lifetime ahead have to suffer the ravages of a destructive malignancy? It is tragic enough with older people who have lived out most of their lives—but a child, that just does not seem fair! We would rather not think about it. But the reality is that cancer is the leading cause of death for persons between the ages of ten and twenty-one. Leukemia, Hodgkin's disease, brain and bone tumors are the most frequently encountered malignancies during this period of life.[10]

Many forms of childhood cancer are incurable. However, more cures are now being achieved and survival rates of those not cured are better than ever before. Because childhood malignancies differ in character from adult cancer, and treatment of children varies at different stages of physiological growth and development, pediatric oncology has become a distinct medical speciality. Centers specializing in research and treatment of childhood malignancies have been established in major cities throughout America. Though few in number, their knowledge of the most effective treatment methods is widely disseminated and available to qualified pediatricians in local areas.

As the life expectancy for children with malignancies increases each year, problems pertaining to the quality of life have become more apparent. The child with cancer may experience confusion, pain, frustration, fear, social isolation and identity crisis. The integrity of the child's family may be threatened by intense emotional trauma, the stress on parent/child relationships, sibling rivalry, intensification of marital problems, and financial crisis.[13] Those around the patients—peers, friends of the family, teachers, health care and service professionals, all have their own problems in relating to them. A sweeping sense of inadequacy heightened by a flood of subjective feelings threatens to paralyze rational thought with counterproductive behavior.

Seven-year-old Tim is a case in point. Tim had gained the reputation of being the number one discipline problem in his school. Every fall the teachers were fearful that he might be assigned to their room. Then the child was diagnosed with incurable cancer. The conflicting feelings of sympathy and anger paralyzed his teacher's interactions with him. She couldn't handle her feelings, so she ignored him. His own anxieties about being "different" were confirmed by his teacher's behavior. In a bid for attention, he began to exhibit aggressive behavior which only intensified the problem. He became the general topic of conversation in the faculty lounge and the object of concern in faculty meetings. It was finally decided that, due to his illness and accompanying behavior, he was gaining nothing from his experience in school. The principal petitioned his parents to remove him from the school system. Even though the child was undergoing medical treatment, he suffered no physical impairment that would severely limit his functional level. He had been caught in a vicious cycle of social stigma often experienced by victims of cancer.

Coping with childhood cancer is difficult for the children and threatening to those around them. Inadequate coping on the part of the family and professional care providers makes matters worse. Appropriate control of emotions and the development of healthy interpersonal relationships alleviate anxiety. Skillful communication and realistic perceptions promote rational decision making that enhances the quality of life for the patient during the illness.

The purpose of this chapter is to assist families experiencing childhood cancer to better understand the psychological and social impact of the illness as well as suggesting guidelines in developing specific coping techniques. I will first discuss the experience from the perspective of preadolescence. Second, cancer and the adolescent will be discussed. Finally, I will focus on the support of the child whose parent has cancer.

Cancer and the Preadolescent

Perception Disparity

Many parents do not think the child who has cancer should be told about it. Great care is taken not to use the word in the child's presence. This is an inappropriate and dangerous reaction for two reasons. First, preadolescent children have not developed intellectually to the point of conceptualized thinking. While they have no well-developed concept of life, death, time, space, or values, they do attach symbolic meanings to illness using fantasy. They may not differentiate cancer from other physical disorders like the common cold or a stomachache. They may not have well-developed defense mechanisms like those employed by adults to avoid painful realities. But they feel pain, disorientation, and frustration as intensely as an adult. Therefore, there is often a disparity of perception between parents and children regarding the experience. Several days before his death a seven-year-old boy nonchalantly described his situation: "I'm going to die, aren't I? I won't get to go fishing next summer, and I won't go into third grade next fall." He had no concept of anything beyond the immediate future. His parents, on the other hand, felt the crushing impact of the loss of their boy who was an extension of their own identity. They felt the laceration of shattered hopes and aspirations of what might have been.

Second, it is dangerous to insulate a child from the truth of a cancer diagnosis because of the insecurity and destruction of trust that evasion precipitates. Cues from nonverbal behavior, hushed conversations, guarded voice inflections and words that are spelled rather than spoken quickly communicate parents' guilt, fear, and grief. Such behavior is anxiety-producing to the child and generates insecurity. If children are to cope with illness, they need a trusting and reassuring relationship with their parents. Parents who remain unaware of the disparity of perception between themselves and the ill child set themselves up for failure.

Guidelines for Effective Coping

Share Feelings—Don't Project Anxieties

When children are suddenly introduced to the strange world of medical procedures, anxiety cues from those around them tell them when to be afraid. Parents are afraid, too. Who wouldn't be? It is better to share these feelings than to suppress them. Mrs. Conner became frightened when her five-year-old daughter became abnormally ill the day after routine treatment for leukemia. She brought her to the clinic in tears. While waiting for the doctor, she rocked her child and cried softly. Examination revealed the reassuring news that her child had only contracted a slight cold. With low resistance due to the illness and treatment, antibiotics were required. The mother confided, "That old demon, fear, gripped me when I saw her get so sick. I was afraid it was serious. I'll be okay now. That's the way I handle fear. I cry and then do what I have to. I guess fear is the worst weapon old Satan has." I suggested to the mother that fear is often a necessary warning of impending danger. Even a slight cold can be highly dangerous to her child at this stage. Her fear had motivated appropriate action resulting in essential medical treatment. The mother replied, "Yes, fear can be helpful—just so you don't hold on to it too long."

All these feelings were expressed in the presence of the child. It was a healthy experience. The mother was letting her child know it is all right to experience and express fear. She was also teaching her an appropriate way to cope.

Too many parents are afraid to let their children know that they are human—afraid to let them see their tears. Hiding unresolved anxiety from children only heightens their insecurity and renders the parent more vulnerable. Children who are ill soon learn to capitalize on the anxieties of those around them. This is not to imply that children are basically diabolical or conniving. In this situation they simply learn to regard manipulation as an easy means to an end. That was little Tim's problem. Prior to his diagnosis his teacher considered him a problem child. Craving attention, he soon learned to deliver the negative behavior she expected of him. Her dislike for the child increased in direct proportion to the frequency of negative behavior. After the diagnosis, his continued negative behavior stimulated conflicting feelings of anger and guilt. The guilt prevented her from reprimanding him. The more she ignored his bids for attention, the more severe his misbehavior became. Soon Tim was more in control than his teacher. Her sympathy, motivated by guilt, became positive reinforcement for his inappropriate behavior. Tim became a mischievous imp. His teacher became an emotional wreck.

Ill children must be taught more appropriate ways of responding to their environment. They cannot learn if the adults around them allow anxiety, fear, and guilt to confuse their interactions.

Just as children can be manipulative so too can they be protective. Wes was a nine-year-old boy with terminal cancer. His parents had always maintained open communication with their children. However, his mother confided that if Wes ever broached the subject of his impending death, she didn't think that she could handle it. One day Wes tested her to see if it was a safe subject. "Mother," he said, "If I ever decided to run away from home and did not go to the clinic for treatments, would I die?"

"Yes," his mother replied, "You need your treatments."
Her verbal communication was simple, honest, direct, and
perfectly appropriate. Her son's reassuring answer, however,
indicates that she nonverbally communicated her anxiety.

"Well, don't worry, Mom. I wasn't planning on running
away." He never brought up the subject again with his parents. However, he later confided to a neighbor that he was not
worried about dying since he "would be with Jesus." Knowing Wes, I am certain he knew that reassurance would get
back to his parents.

Include the Child in Decision Making

One way of teaching ill children how to respond appropriately to their strange new environment and work through
anxiety is to include them in making decisions about medical
treatment by presenting realistic and understandable options
to them. Even when the child is too young to participate
intelligently in the conversation, the importance of his parents
and the health care team modeling a rational decision-making
process cannot be overestimated. Children should witness this
process and then have decisions explained in terms that they
can understand.

In short, children should not be excluded from decision
making. Exclusion confirms their anxieties over being "different" and stimulates their imagination to exaggerate the situation out of perspective with reality. Children should be
given information that is appropriate to their needs and their
ability to understand.

Encourage Responsibility Commensurate with Ability

Living with illness is a learning experience for both child
and parents. Children have their own level of needs for orientation to the experience given their emotional state and stage
of development. As we have observed, parents must not complicate the child's adjustment by disparity of perception or
projection of their own anxieties. Children cannot learn if
they are not given a measure of responsibility commensurate

with their ability. They have a right to some degree of control over their environment. Unless that right is granted, they will have no investment in the treatment program and may tend to be uncooperative. By being taught responsibility they will learn to respect the rights and authority of others. Children should be given a straightforward explanation of what is to be done and why. They should be informed of the respective roles of those involved. Then they will know what they can expect of others and what is expected of them as well. They must know, unequivocally, the rules of the game and the pleasures and pains of participation.

Contrived fantasies are a poor substitute for plain truth. They are confusing, misleading, and destructive. Leukemia by any other name is just as deadly. Even though the technical name may be hidden from the child, as symptoms increase the severity of the disease will be self-evident. A shot is a shot and children don't like needles. To say it won't hurt is a lie and an insult to the intelligence. Better to say, "This is going to hurt for a second, but we have already talked about why it is necessary. I know that you can be brave." Trust children with a clear-cut responsibility and they will usually keep their part of the bargain. Children haven't yet learned the adult game of copping out. Leave it to the kids. They will usually come through. It is written, "a little child shall lead them."

This is true in family relationships as well as in medical treatment procedures. The greatest temptation for parents is to pamper the ill child. Young Wes' parents initially found themselves so overwhelmed with grief that they set no limits on his behavior. This lasted about three days. He became as unhappy with himself as they were with him. He needed limits in order to clarify his role and maintain self-respect as well as the respect of his brothers and sisters.

His parents learned that if the way you are handling things doesn't get rid of the knot in the pit of your stomach, you must be doing something wrong. It is time to speak up about those feelings—"Look here, we love you, and it hurts us when you feel sick, but certain behavior is unacceptable. Cool it!" Children usually appreciate knowing their limits. It confirms the fact that their parents care.

The security that authority brings a child should not be underestimated. Wes died at home by choice. He enjoyed life and faced death with equanimity because his parents entrusted him with appropriate responsibility.

Responsibility and reassurance are not always imparted by words. Often our strongest feelings are expressed in silence. A story from the experiences of Elizabeth Kübler-Ross illustrates this. A boy dying in an oxygen tent called for the nurse. "What will happen if the hospital catches fire while I am in this oxygen tent?" he asked. "Don't worry," the nurse reassured him. "That is not going to happen." She picked up non-verbal cues from the child that led her to share her concerns with her supervisor. The supervisor concluded that the boy needed to talk about his imminent death.

The nurse confessed that she couldn't cope with that. I think most of us could empathize with her. The supervisor agreed to talk with the boy. "I understand that you have some concern for your safety," she began.

"Yes," he queried, "what will happen to me if the hospital catches fire while I am in this oxygen tent?" She slipped under the tent, laying the upper part of her body beside the child, embracing him.

"Would this help?" she asked. The reassurance of benevolent authority inspired trust which enabled the boy to freely share his concerns about dying. No words of reassurance were necessary.

Cancer and the Adolescent

Many of the problems observed in children also apply to adolescents. Adolescents have the additional stress of being at the difficult stage between childhood and adulthood when they are beginning to think in concepts, develop a sense of identity, and formulate value structures. They are reluctant to trade the freedom of childhood for adult responsibilities even though they desire adult privileges.

Cancer strikes the adolescent with shattering impact. Much significant work in adolescent oncology has been accomplished by Charlene Holt, M.D. She states, "Though sufficiently mature to appreciate the implication of the diagnosis and prognosis, the adolescent has not yet completed the personality integration or has fully evolved adult defense mechanism which might enable him to adjust successfully to the knowledge of his illness." [10] Much of the material in this section is based on the work of Dr. Holt and her colleagues at St. Jude's Hospital.

Problems of the adolescent cancer patient fall into four major categories: alteration of self-concept, alteration of body image, difficulty in interpersonal relationships, and interference with future plans.

Alteration of Self-Esteem

Peer relationships are most important to adolescents. Feelings of being "different" when "belonging" is important supersedes the fear of death and may stimulate patients to attempt to conceal their illness. Various coping mechanisms are employed in order to preserve self-esteem.

Denial is one mechanism often employed by adolescent patients. A 16-year-old patient spent his summers working as a buckaroo. On long cattle drives he spent weeks at a time riding, roping, and camping out under the stars. His malignancy was responsive to chemotherapy with a high probability of cure. His physician was puzzled to discover the medication was not achieving the expected response. The boy finally confided, "I haven't been taking my medication during cattle drives because I don't want the fellows to know that I am sick and think I am a weakling."

Overcompensation is another mechanism employed by adolescent patients. As soon after treatment as possible the overcompensating patient will become abnormally intent on excelling in some competitive field in order to maintain his self-esteem. This is a healthy adolescent reaction to a perceived or actual defect. Although strenuous physical activity may in some cases enhance the risk of accidents and injuries, most pediatric oncologists think it is worth the risk because of the quality of life enjoyed by the patient.

Some adolescents cope by *intellectualizing*. They become avid readers and ask penetrating questions about the illness, treatment and outcome. This is a healthy method of coping since intellectual mastery of knowledge decreases anxiety. Such questions should be answered with honesty and reassurance. One patient said, "I ask questions so that I will know what to tell others." Finding answers helped her with her underlying question, "How will this make me different and change my life?"

Anger is a very prevalent means of coping for adolescent patients. Adolescents are beginning to think in terms of time and values. Although they may not be making long-range plans, they resent any change of plans for the immediate future. Jay's father and mother had been divorced for several years. Jay had lived with his mother, whose rigid religious convictions had placed severe restrictions on his activities. At age 14 Jay moved in with his father. He was ecstatic over the prospect of being allowed to play football for the first time in his life. On a routine physical examination by the team's physician, a malignancy was discovered. Jay was justifiably angry. His anger over being washed out for the season superseded his fear of death or the sterility that might result from illness and treatment.

A patient's anger may be directed toward parents, peers or the health care team. A cardinal rule for interacting with patients is that they all have a right to their feelings. Expressing anger is therapeutic. However, excessive or abusive anger is inappropriate and need not be accepted. Continued acceptance only reinforces the behavior and doesn't help the adolescent develop more productive alternatives.

Regression is another coping mechanism employed by ado-

lescent patients. A 20-year-old man was diagnosed with incurable malignancy. He had excelled in athletics and had
considered becoming professional. He was engaged to be married at the time of diagnosis. Both his mother and fiancee
became solicitous to the point of competing for his attention.
The young man found himself in the dilemma of choosing
between them. He broke the engagement, explaining to his
fiancee that, since their future together was limited by his illness, a continued investment in the relationship would only
result in heartbreak. He regressed to childhood, accepting his
mother's constant company and care in exchange for his
independence.

Alteration of the Body

Physical changes resulting from treatment accentuate the
normal rapid body change of the adolescent. Hair loss resulting from chemotherapy is one of the most difficult adjustments for adolescents. Girls can wear wigs less noticeably than
boys. Being bald as a teenager is difficult. Excessive weight
gain resulting from drugs is another problem experienced by
the adolescent. Amputation of a limb often precipitates fear of
being unacceptable. Patients mourn for the limb much the
same as they would the death of a friend.

Difficulty in Interpersonal Relationships

To the average adolescent, dependency equals weakness.
The fear of being weak has impact on interpersonal relationships. Frankness of peers is difficult for patients who are
already emotionally compromised by their illness. The fear of
rejection often causes them to become infuriated at sympathy
offered by family and friends.

The patient's peers often react to their own strange feelings
about the illness and not to the patient personally. This becomes confusing to the patient, arousing ambivalent feelings,
and threatening the relationship.

Guilt feelings of parents may result in overindulgence of

the patient. Overprotective parents can make it difficult for the patient to accept the illness and treatment.

Interference with Future Plans

Adolescents who know their illness is life-threatening wonder about the future just as do adults. Seeking reassurance, they may ask questions that may imply longevity. They may ask, "Should I apply for college?" The underlying question may be, "Will I live long enough to finish college?" Patients who achieve remission often express concern about recurrence of the disease. Loss of reproductive ability is a definite risk with some forms of treatment. To a female, the loss of ability to reproduce, like loss of hair or limb, may mean loss of femininity and may result in alteration of self-esteem. It is a harsh reality for which there are no answers to soften the blow. It is a difficult problem to answer these questions without either destroying the adolescent's hope, or encouraging false optimism.

Guidelines for Interaction

Be Honest

Above all else the adolescent patient must be treated with honesty. Games of evasion are lies. Lies destroy trust and violate one's dignity and sense of propriety. I have seen cases in which parents chose not to reveal the diagnosis to their child. There is no way to hide the reality of cancer forever. When the truth was learned, the patients could never trust their parents again. Nothing is more painful to an adolescent than to face death in the loneliness of distrust. No guilt is more severe than that felt after seeing to one's own child die knowing that trust was lost forever.

Allow Freedom—Expect Responsibility

Interest and trust from adults yields responsibility and trust from adolescents. Adolescents are beginning to develop adult concepts. When faced with a cancer diagnosis, they are confronting an adult crisis. Therefore they should be treated as adults. To do otherwise destroys self-esteem.

Kevin was 13 when diagnosed with a tumor of the brain stem. He possessed a near genius IQ. He was an avid reader, prolific writer and an accomplished athlete. His prognosis was frightening—a degenerative process of motor function, general paralysis, ultimate death. Confrontation of Kevin's plight disarmed most of the health care team. He was such a cute, red-haired "Charlie Brown," and it was so easy to pamper him. But pampering only spoiled him by reinforcing dependency and regression.

Kevin's parents are separated. His mother had to work and care for the other children in a town distant from the treatment center. She realized Kevin's constant care was beyond her physical capability. Though it was difficult for her to part with her son, she sought his father's assistance. Kevin's father is a wise and sensitive man, devoted to his son. He quit his job in order to spend all of his time with Kevin in his remaining years. At home, when Kevin asked for something his father would respond, "You want it. Go get it." It was not easy for Kevin. It was even more difficult for his father. Once Kevin fell and broke a chair. He cried and apologized. His father comforted him, "That's okay son. We can always buy another chair. Your self-respect is priceless. I am proud of the way you keep going."

Kevin's father knew his son's limits and never pushed him beyond them. He worked with the boy to keep his mind and body active. He encouraged peer relationships in order to enhance Kevin's social skills. Largely due to his father's expectation of responsibility, Kevin remained alive and functional far beyond the initial medical prognosis.

Parental support is essential to the adolescent, but it is not enough. They need healthy interactions with others. When Kevin was 16, his illness had progressed to the point that he could no longer be cared for at home. He was admitted to a rehabilitation hospital. The staff immediately fell in love with him. Their love often took the form of pampering. Kevin's progress was hindered. His self-esteem deteriorated and he went into a depression. One evening at dinner Kevin met Manny Shaw. Manny is an old Idaho rancher whose avocation is playing the fiddle. Several days after suffering a paralytic stroke, Manny called for his fiddle. He positioned the fingers of his paralyzed hand on the strings. With his good hand maneuvering the bow, he entertained the entire hospital to the strains of the "Wabash Cannonball."

Manny has hopes as high as the Sawtooth Mountains outside his front window, and a sensitivity as deep as the Snake River Canyon. That evening at dinner Manny sat across from Kevin watching him chase the peas around his plate. Kevin could no longer grasp anything with his fingers. His fork was strapped to his hand. Manny suggested he stick the fork directly into the peas rather than trying to roll them onto his fork. Kevin managed a sickly smile from a depressed posture and continued to roll the peas around the plate. With a voice that could be heard across town, Manny shouted, "Stab 'em, dammit, or starve!" Kevin's eyes lit up, his shoulders straightened and a broad smile broke out like the morning sun. That was the first time anyone other than his father had talked to him like a man. He stabbed his peas and ate a big dinner.

Through honesty, trust, and responsibility in his human relationships, Kevin lived the equivalent of fifty years in sixteen. The day he died, his grieving father managed to smile and say, "Despite Kevin's illness, these last three years have been the best three years of our lives."

Children of Cancer Patients

The child whose parent has cancer should be treated in much the same manner as the pediatric patient. Parental feelings should be shared. The children should not be excluded from the experience, and should be given information appropriate to their age and level of understanding.

Some years ago a young radiology technologist came to me for career counseling. She wanted to leave the diagnostic branch of radiology and enter the cancer treatment modality of radiation therapy. I suggested to her that working constantly with cancer patients can be emotionally depleting, and I asked about her motives. She told me that her father had become ill when she was a small child. Her parents chose not to tell her that he had cancer. As the illness progressed, he underwent radical personality changes. She was confused and frustrated. Her ardent love for him changed to hatred. "Once," she reported, "I wished he would die. Then he did die. If they had only told me. . . . I would have done so many things differently. There are so many things left unsaid that he can never hear."

Contrast that with the experience of Gary, a 36-year-old father of five. Gary lived only two years after his diagnosis. During his illness he reported:

> I think the kids today are looking for truth. They don't want to hear about Santa Claus and the good tooth fairy. They want facts. So we told our children what I have . . . the fact that I have lung cancer, that I can't be cured, but I am not giving up. I don't term us a religious family, but we believe there is a God to turn to for help in making the best of what you've got and what you've had. I have heard my children cry and sob in their beds at night for daddy, and I've heard them pray for me. Whenever we need to talk about it, we do. I think it has made them stronger.

Gary's children were young when he died. The reality of his death didn't have its full impact for several years. When they began the grieving process, the open communication they enjoyed with their father helped them develop coping skills that enabled them to maintain stability and a sense of fulfillment they may not otherwise have achieved.

Conclusion

Helping children cope with cancer in themselves or a loved one is a heavy responsibility. Most of us feel inadequate for the job. Perhaps it will help if we can look upon life as a trust. Life is not of our own contrivance, it is a gift. Every young parent, upon the miracle of birth of each child, has felt a deep sense of gratitude for the gift of life. In *Living with Dying*, Dr. Glen W. Davidson states, "If I accept life as a gift, then dying is part of the given." [3] When we lose sight of the Giver, we cannot see beyond ourselves and our own experience. We begin to think that everything depends on us, and become imprisoned within the walls of our own anxiety and fear of inadequacy. Trusting the Giver of life enables us to relax and admit we are human. Parents who are free enough to be honest and share their feelings with their children discover that kids are people too. Then they are free to face life together and build relationships that can endure anything— even death. The prayer of a young mother whose only son had leukemia demonstrates that trust:

> Dear God, we don't pretend to understand why our little Jerry has to suffer, but we thank you for the gift of his life for whatever time we can have him. Help us to use that time wisely and invest ourselves in his guidance and care. When the time comes to give him up, it will hurt us deeply. Give us grace to freely commend him to your keeping. Amen.

7

Cancer:
The End or
a Beginning?

For most people a diagnosis of cancer means the beginning of the end. To many, cancer means death, pain, suffering, contamination, ostracism, dependency, and abandonment. The grotesque shapes anxiety gives to cancer can be overwhelming and disorienting. So overwhelming are the implications that some choose to deny reality. That may be an appropriate defense temporarily, but we have already discussed the destructive effects of perpetual denial. When patients and their families are able to keep their feelings in touch with reality, they discover that cancer is not the end, but a new beginning. They discover that cancer patients are not lepers, nor need they be classified as victims. They are people no better or worse—or worse off—than anyone else. They discover meaning in suffering. Through their suffering they find new meaning in life and see death as a natural process of life.

Cancer Patients Are Normal People

The physical changes along with the overt and implied ostracism experienced by the person with cancer usually precipitate an identity crisis. When the patients come to the realization that, physical changes and societal reactions not-

101

withstanding, they are the same person they were prior to diagnosis, then they have made the first step toward recovery —self-acceptance.

Acceptance in the eyes of God is the primary quest of every major religion. Each has its own set of doctrines, regulations, and rituals through which its celebrants can achieve acceptance. The Christians have a word for it—*grace*. Which of us, as parents, would make our love for our children something they must earn? We may put contingencies on our approval, but never on our love.

The physical disharmony and social ostracism experienced by people with cancer often causes a temporary identity crisis. When anxieties are resolved by reality, the patients then understand that cancer is a physical illness, not a personality disorder, so they need not feel guilty, unacceptable, or "different." The cancer experience may lead to new self-discovery and new insight.

Meaning in Suffering

Famous men who are winners enjoy the plaudits of the crowd. Famous men who lose must struggle to publicly accept defeat with at least the appearance of grace. The pain of defeat can be seen behind the forced smile of the losing candidate as he makes his concession speech. Some, embittered by defeat, sink into anonymity. Others, whose faith gives them the freedom to fail, learn how to turn defeat into victory. Hubert Humphrey was that kind of man. He humbled his political adversaries by never speaking a bitter word. With dignity he productively supported those to whom he had lost. In his final days, he inspired an empathetic nation as he demonstrated how one can lose a battle with cancer but win the war of life. Walter Mondale echoed the thoughts of Humphrey's friends as well as his adversaries when he eulogized, "He taught us how to win and how to lose. He taught us how to live and finally, he taught us how to die."

Those perceptive and sensitive enough to find meaning in their suffering leave the rest of us a legacy of life beyond measure. The names used in this chapter are not fictitious. They are real people. Their message to us is part of their lives and should bear their true names.

The initial suffering of most cancer patients is not with physical pain, but the psychological trauma of the diagnosis. Initially any physical pain is temporary. As the disease progresses there can be periods of intense physical pain and suffering that can only be fully appreciated by another patient.

These periods of pain can precipitate a temporary disorientation. Patients and families who thought they had made satisfactory adjustment may find themselves again experiencing doubt, fear, anger, and frustration. The daughter of a patient describes this experience:

> I'm getting angry. Angry like the little girl that was just pushed aside because she didn't have the right change to get into the movie and was turned back. Angry like when you reach as hard as you can for the top shelf and all the boxes fall on your head. Frustrated anger like someone has tied my hands behind my back and my nose itches and I can't scratch it. Hurt anger like when everyone else got a Christmas present and I did not. I am angry at helplessness and grief. All one can do now is give with love.

Apparently this woman has decided to direct her anger and frustration in constructive ways.

In search of meaning in their suffering, many patients and families try to find some object of blame for the cancer. It is usually an object outside and away from themselves like a doctor who was not alert and did not take the patient's earliest complaints seriously. Those who become preoccupied with this search usually do not mature from the experience, and do great damage to themselves with their paranoia.

By contrast, patients who decide to counter the physical

destruction of cancer with a positive attitude and constructive behavior, will always find meaning in suffering. Margaret Wilcox is a case in point. When initially diagnosed, it was believed that her disease had been caught early enough so that she could be completely cured. It was to be a straightforward procedure: two simple radium implants followed by surgery. Then surgery revealed widespread malignancy. The new prognosis was death within six months to one year.

After the initial shock Margaret said, "This is the most important experience of my life. I don't intend to waste a moment of it." And she didn't. She wrote and published a family history and traveled around the world to visit her children between courses of chemotherapy. Margaret had every reason to feel angry, frustrated, and bitter. She could have resigned herself to six miserable months and died in lonely dejection. Instead, she chose to find meaning in her suffering, lived three fulfilling years, and died a happy woman.

New Faith in Life

The sweeping adjustments precipitated by cancer cannot be underestimated. Adjusting to the probability of living the rest of one's life with a chronic, incurable illness is no small matter. Changes in life-style, long periods of treatment and side effects, periodic hospitalization, the potential loss of rewarding activities and life itself—all can make one stop and wonder, "What is the use? What is life all about?" People confronted with those realities begin to search for something they can rely on in life to carry them through death.

Glee Hohnbaum has been coping with cancer for years. She expresses her faith in herself, her family, and in God:

> Because of our faith, death itself is not a frightening prospect. While I may be under the age at which some people die, I have perhaps lived more in my forty-three years than some people who live to be eighty. Life has been, and still is, good to me.

Just because we've been told I have a terminal disease does not mean it is now time to lie down and wait. As long as physically possible, I've tried to live as we always have. I found it necessary to quit my job, because, as a result of my medication I have a lowered resistance to other diseases and was absent too much to be effective. I continue to do as much as possible at home. My husband, uncomplainingly, does what I cannot manage. There were some loose ends I needed to take care of, which is an advantage of knowing one's disease is terminal. I have usually handled most of our family bookkeeping, so I needed to discuss this more with my husband, so he'll be able to take it over when I can't do it. We double-checked our wills and considered memorial services.

How do we cope with a terminal disease? We are supportive of each other. We help others to accept it, and we accept help from others. We look to God for guidance, and we thank him for the love which we have. We live today without fearing tomorrow.

A person's faith is an individual matter. One articulate patient states, "Some people are born with faith; some acquire it from upbringing and experiences over the years; some never get it at all; and some do only when they confront the fact that there is nothing—absolutely nothing—left but faith in some power beyond their own to help them. I can't tell anyone how to acquire faith, but I can affirm that it helps people who have cancer." Another patient said:

I don't pretend to understand all I have heard ministers say about faith, redemption, and atonement. I'm not sure I know what those words mean. But when I think of Christ, who he was, his purpose, and his despair in the garden—somehow it gives me strength and meaning for my own Gethsemane.

Not everyone has a formalized religious faith, but everyone has faith in something. We can be assured the sun will rise and set everyday, that season will follow season, and that the law of gravity cannot be repealed by Congress. For the most part, we can rely on our family, friends, and co-workers. Richard Niebuhr goes one step further in asserting:

> It is a curious and inescapable fact about our lives, of which we all become aware at some time or another, that we cannot live without a cause, without some object of devotion, some center of worth, something on which we rely for meaning. In this sense all men have faith . . . we never merely believe that life is worth living, but always think of it as made worth living by something on which we rely. And this being, whatever it be, may be properly termed our god.[22]

People with cancer, facing the prospect of chronic illness and probable death, find themselves searching for that object of trust or faith that will give meaning and coherence to their lives and significance to their suffering. As surely as night follows day, when we are confronted with our own mortality, we are abruptly faced with the choice of continuing our cherished little games and evasive maneuvers with reality, or getting on with the real business of living. The happiest, most courageous, best adjusted people I have known are those with cancer who have reassessed life's priorities and have taught me the true meaning of trust and effective interdependence. They have found new faith in life.

A Perspective on Dying

Just as people with cancer often find new faith in life, they usually develop a new perspective on dying. Dying is an experience we all must face whether it comes from cancer, heart disease, or a Mack truck. People confronted with a life-threatening illness, like cancer, think of death in more imminent terms than the rest of us. When one is going through the process of dying, he searches for some meaning, some cohesive concept or power to maintain his equilibrium. Those who seek usually find it, and not without some help from others. Lois Jaffe, a 47-year-old mother-wife-educator-social worker-acute leukemia patient discribes her own search:

> . . . at every juncture where I have been helped to face my impending death, help has come from a sensitivity and care that others have demonstrated regarding a respect for my life, rather than a despair over my death. Before I used to see life as a straight line which was cut off at the end. Now I see life as a circle of fulfilled life, it equals infinity.[21]

As people approach death, they often discover that the gods in which they have placed their faith, cherished and meaningful as they have been, are transitory and unable to save them from the ultimate frustration of meaninglessness. We must all face what Niebuhr calls "the twilight of the gods." It occurs when we realize that all our ideas, all our causes, all the beings on which we relied to save us from worthlessness are doomed to pass. Our loved ones can hold our hand as we stand at death's door, and they can wave good-bye, but we must go through the door alone.

Through fifteen years as a pastor and six years as counselor to cancer patients and their families, I have seen many people die. For a long time I felt helpless and inadequate because I could only accompany people to death's door. Then I discovered that was an ego trip. They did not really need me once they arrived at the door. All those feelings I had were a projection of my own anxieties. Most of the patients had found a comfort neither I nor anyone else could give. Even patients who have expressed fear of death can get to the door and find peace and contentment. It is as though all the experiences of this life have subtly prepared them for this moment and have given them assurance that the best is yet to come.

The story of Elaine, a 14-year-old girl with leukemia, best illustrates the strength of collective life experience and the dimension of faith that helps many through the twilight of their gods.

Elaine had never really known her father. He had been committed to a mental hospital when she was a small girl. Her mother was employed as a nurses' aide and struggled to support three of her four children. Elaine had two brothers, twenty and fifteen years old, and a sister thirteen. Her family shared a small farm with a couple in their mid-thirties.

The day Elaine's illness was finally diagnosed, the attending physician explained to her and her mother the recommended treatment and prognosis:

> Leukemia is a disease of the blood. In order to live, we must have healthy blood. Right now you have more leukemic cells than healthy cells in your blood. That means there are bad guys in your bloodstream fighting the good guys. Right now the bad guys have the upper hand. I'm going to give you some chemicals to help the good guys defend themselves. The chemicals will have some strong reactions. You will lose your hair. You will be nauseated for a few hours after your treatments, and you may get some canker sores in your mouth. We can get you a wig before you lose your hair, so your friends will never know the difference. We can give you medication to reduce your nausea and ointment for the canker sores. All of these reactions are temporary. Even though they are disturbing they are necessary to beat those bad guys who are destroying your blood. When the medicine takes effect, the bad guys will disappear, and you will be able to function normally. We call that a remission. At some point in the future the medicine will no longer be effective and the bad guys will win. All of us must die sometime. The difference be-

tween you and me is, because of your illness, your
realization of that fact is greater than mine.

Elaine contemplated awhile and replied, "My main goal
right now is to compete next summer in the Snake River
Stampede. I've been elected queen of my riding club. I don't
know if I can win, but I want to represent my club well."
The physician assured her that was a realistic goal, and prom-
ised to have her ready to ride in the stampede.

Elaine was a quiet child and talked very little, especially to
adults. She loved animals, and had a special way with horses.
A soft and reassuring word from Elaine to a frightened horse,
and it would understand everything she was saying. She
soon learned to transfer some of her savvy with animals to
her interpersonal relationships. Her physician helped with
this by suggesting she invite her brothers and sister to accompany her to the clinic. He had her explain the nature of her
illness and treatment to them. In this way she grew to understand it better, learned to express herself and gained self-confidence.

Elaine responded well to treatment and did achieve a remission. Life was going well for her. She was a happy, well-ad-
justed young lady growing up and exploring new worlds in
spite of her illness. A neighbor had given her a beautiful
mare with foal. It was one of the happiest days of her life
when her mare presented her with a healthy colt. Early each
morning Elaine could be seen standing at the fence, silhouetted
against the rising sun, calling to her mare. The mare would
answer, and gallop, with the colt at her side, to nuzzle her
mistress. One morning the mare failed to answer the call. The
colt came to her alone. Vaulting the fence, Elaine found her
mare lying dead in the pasture. The loss was acute, but Elaine
accepted it with equanimity. She nursed the colt from a bottle
till he was able to eat on his own.

Not long after the mare's death, Elaine's mother underwent
surgery and died unexpectedly. Permanent foster care was arranged with the young couple with whom they had been

sharing the farm. Tex and Becky cared for the children as
though they were their own.

The time of Elaine's big day at the rodeo was approach-
ing. Perfecting riding skills for the queen's competition
occupied most of her time. The girls were required to participate in the grand parade five evenings, competing for high
honors. All the other competitors were older than Elaine
and looked svelte and comely in their form fitting costumes.
Elaine with her freckles and pigtails looked more like the
mascot than a queen. She knew her chances of winning were
remote, but she was happy for the privilege of competing.
She and her foster parents had chosen not to inform the
judges of her illness. It might bias their decision. To those
of us who watched her ride that night she was the queen,
regardless of the judge's decision. There was good reason
for additional anxiety as we watched her daring ride. There
were indications that Elaine was no longer in remission. A
traumatic injury could have precipitated a fatal hemorrhage.

Elaine was thrilled. The dream of a lifetime for her had
come true. The next day she returned to the clinic for her
check-up. With great elation and dancing eyes she said to
Dr. Steuart, "Since I was able to ride in the stampede, the
next thing I want to do is take a tour of the Holy Land
with my minister." He replied, "I am sorry Elaine, but you
are no longer in remission. I think you know what that
means."

During the next several weeks she became weaker and
was admitted to the hospital. Prior to her admission she
divided her possessions among her brothers and sister.
Elaine was in the hospital just a few days. On the day of
her death she asked her foster father to lie down beside her
and said to him, "I don't think I ever told you how much
I love you or appreciate all of the things you have done for
my family. Please stay with me today. I will need you until
it is over." Those of us who stood by her bed experienced
the redemptive quality of suffering innocence.

Elaine's death was a tragedy, but who would say her life

was wasted? She learned, as all of us should learn, that death is an event in the natural process of life. Pre-occupation with fear of death only detracts from the quality of life. The quality of one's life enhanced by the integrity of human relationships gives momentum to the journey through the experience of death.

Living Legends

It isn't necessary for one to die to achieve victory in the battle with cancer. There is a growing army of people who have overcome cancer and live to share a fuller dimension of meaning in life. Some are famous like Shirley Temple Black, John Wayne, Betty Ford, Happy Rockefeller, Frank Church, and Tracy Andrus. Others are unknown beyond their small circle of acquaintances. Kathryn Simpson was in the latter group. With double-edged humor that belies her saintly stature she tells her story:

> Dr. Moschel was a great doctor for me to start out with because he never talked down to me, never patronized me. He also gave me a few candles with which to light the darkness into which he had helped lead me. For instance, concerning my prognosis he said, "I have a feeling about you. I think you are one of the survivors in life." And possibly thereby helped trigger the fight to recover and lead a normal life. At one point, when I was asking him about my survival chances he did discuss them briefly, mostly by saying "you have access to the same statistics I have and you can read." But then he looked right at me and said, "Of course, I can't guarantee you will live long enough to die from cancer either."
>
> For the first few days after surgery I was kept pretty heavily sedated so my recollections are hazy. However, a few thoughts did come through loud

and clear. One was the remembrance of discussion a group of us had several years earlier when we were discussing how we would prefer to die. Each person at the table said they preferred to be killed instantly, but I said, "Not me. I prefer to die of cancer or something so I'd know ahead of time. I will have things to take care of and my life to get in order and I prefer to know ahead of time." My husband, Jim, agreed with me. So I thought, OK kid, you asked for this, now how are you going to handle it? Are you going to be equal to the task? So I lay there thinking about other women I had known who had faced the problem. I thought about the women I had known who had had breast cancer and died. Then I thought about women I had known who had had breast cancer and might just as well have died. Then I thought about Ann. Ann was the mother of a friend of ours who lived across the street from us. Ann had had a breast removed several years before. But Ann golfed; Ann hosted all of the neighborhood coffee hours; Ann carted her grandchildren around town; Ann was always available as a fourth for bridge, and it wasn't until I really stopped to think about her that I realized how much I really observed Ann. So Ann was to be my rallying cry.

It was also during this time I realized the single most important thing in my life was my own personal relationship with God. I loved my family and they were important to me, but not as important as my God. I am grateful to my husband for many things (just putting up with me being one of them) but I am perhaps most grateful to him for bringing me into his church. Jim was a Lutheran and I found his church fitted me to a tee. It has been my rock.

Have I learned anything from my experience?

> Well, I've at least observed some things. I am
> very grateful God allowed me to walk through
> his beautiful world for a time. I have enjoyed it
> immensely. I have been fortunate in that I have
> met many wonderful people in my walk through
> life.
>
> God has been very good to me. One of the ways
> I have been blessed is that whenever I really needed
> help, someone was always there to take my hand
> and say, "I will walk a way with you."
>
> Of course, I have one other problem. I'm a
> born optimist. I have never gone to bed a night in
> my life that I wasn't sure things would be better
> tomorrow. So really I don't know if I can give up
> the fight, even if I try.

Since the time Kathryn wrote those words she has had a total hip replacement subsequent to a pathological fracture resulting from metastasis to the bone. Although she had been on maintenance chemotherapy for years, medication was withdrawn for the surgery in order to allow her blood count to improve. Since there was no evidence of tumor progression subsequent to surgery she was allowed to remain off treatment. At the time of this writing, she has been without treatment for six months with no sign of disease progression. She has no illusions regarding cure, but is thankful for each day without symptoms. Her town built a park and named it in her honor. The landscaping was rushed in order for Katy to see it before she died. Now she says the shrubbery has grown up and she's still around. "I don't try to explain it," says Katy, "I just tell it like it is." She is now in her thirteenth year with cancer.

Conclusion

Those of us involved in the cancer experience—patient, family, clinician—confront the basic issues of life, its quality and its meaning. As we become professionally and personally involved with people who have cancer we learn basic truths never read in theological dissertations or psychological explanations. We learn that courage and character is cultivated, not inherited. We learn that we can confront and conquer fear, even when we are afraid. We learn the meaning of interdependence and what it means in the human family to be members one of another.

When the good die young we are prone to cry, "What a waste!" When the old depart we miss their wisdom. But people who have learned to cope with the cancer crisis teach us that if the moments of life are not wasted it matters not whether we die soon or late. For those who are left behind it hurts. But we begin to understand something of the positive impact, the therapeutic value and the redemptive quality of suffering innocence. We learn from them the meaning of being at one with oneself, with others and with the cohesive power behind the universe.

Albert Schweitzer said it well in his *The Quest of the Historical Jesus:*

> He comes to us as One unknown, without a name,
> as of old, by the lake, He came to those men who
> knew Him not. He speaks the same word: "Follow
> thou me," and sets us to the tasks which he has to
> fulfill in our time. He commands. And to those
> who obey Him, whether they be wise or simple,
> He will reveal Himself in the toils, the conflicts, the
> sufferings which they shall pass through in his fel-
> lowship, and, as an ineffable mystery, they shall
> learn in their own experience Who He is.

Those who experience this inner peace and harmony have truly learned how to live—not just survive. Their experience echoes the truth spoken by St. John:

> The light still shines in the darkness,
> and the darkness has never put it out.
>
> (JOHN 1:5)

References

1. Brightman, Edgar Sheffield, *A Philosophy of Religion.* Englewood Cliffs, NJ: Prentice-Hall, 1956.
2. Coursey, Katherine, B.S., Dawson, John, M.Div., Luce, J. K., M.D., "Comparative Anxiety Levels of Cancer Patients and Families," *ASCO Proceedings,* 1975.
3. Davidson, Glen W., *Living with Dying.* Minneapolis: Augsburg, 1975.
4. Frank, Jerome D., *Persuasion and Healing.* Baltimore and London: Johns Hopkins University Press, 1973.
5. Friedman, M.D., Rosenman, Hay H., M.D., *Type A Behavior and Your Heart.* Greenwich, CT.: Fawcett, 1974.
6. Harkness, Georgia, *Understanding the Christian Faith.* Nashville: Abingdon.
7. Holmes, Thomas, M.D., "How Change Can Make Us Ill," *Stress: Blue Print for Health,* Blue Cross Association, Vol. XXV, Number 1, Chicago: 1974.
8. Holmes, T. Stephenson and Holmes, Thomas H., "Short-term Intrusion into the Life Style Routine," *Journal of Psychosomatic Research,* Vol. 14, pp. 121 to 132. (Verification: Separation and Depression AAAS, 1973, p. 184.)
9. Holmes, Thomas L. and Rahe, Richard H., "The Social Readjustment Rating Scale," *Journal of Psychosomatic Research,* Vol. 11, pp. 213-218. (Verification: Separation and Depression AAAS 1973, p. 184).

10. Holt, Charlene P., "Psychological Aspects of the Management of Adolescents with Malignancy," MCV Quarterly 7 (3): 112-119, 1971.

11. Kelly, Orville E., *Make Today Count*. New York: Delacorte, 1975.

12. Kübler-Ross, Elizabeth, *On Death and Dying*. New York: MacMillan, 1972.

13. Lansky, Shirley B., "Update on Psychosocial Problems in Childhood Cancer," *Cancer Control for the Professional* (Vol. 3, No. 4), The American Cancer Society: Kansas Division, Inc., Topeka, Kansas: July/August 1976.

14. Luce, James K., Dawson, J. J., "Quality of Life," *Seminars in Oncology*, December 1975.

15. Pelletier, Kenneth R., Ph.D., "Mind as Healer—Mind as Slayer," *Psychology Today*, Feb., 1977, p. 35.

16. Symonton, Carl O., "Belief and Management of the Emotional Aspects of Malignancy," *Journal of Transpersonal Psychology*, Vol. VII, No. 1, 1975. Box 4437, Stanford, California 94305.

17. Toffler, Alvin, *Future Shock*. New York: Bantam, 1970.

18. Weatherhead, Leslie D., *The Christian Agnostic*. Nashville: Abingdon, 1975.

19. Weisman, Avery, M.D., Worden, J. William, Ph.D., "The Existential Plight in Cancer: Significance of the First 100 Days," *Internal Journal Psychiatry in Medicine*, Vol. 7 (1), Baywood Publishing Co., Inc.: 1976.

20. Engel, George L., "Sudden and Rapid Death During Psychological Stress," *Annals of Internal Medicine*, Vol. 74, No. 5, May 1971.

21. Jaffe, Lois, "Making Time Count," keynote address to *Quality of Life Conference*. Pittsburgh: Mercy Hospital, November 1974.

22. Niebuhr, H. Richard, "Faith in Gods and in God," *Motive*, December 1943.

Practical Aids
for Patient and Family

The American Cancer Society
777 Third Avenue
New York, New York 10017
212-371-2900

ACS is primarily engaged in producing cancer education resources and providing support for research. Individual patient support programs include Reach to Recovery, for the mastectomized patient, and Ostomy Clubs which provide educational and emotional support for the ostomy patient and spouse. Some state chapters provide limited transportation funds for patients. For information contact your local ACS representative.

Leukemia Society of America, Inc.
211 East 43rd Street
New York, New York 10017

The Leukemia Society provides limited financial support to victims of leukemia in states where a chapter has been organized.

Candlelighters
123 "C" Street, S.E.
Washington, D.C. 20003
202-544-1696

Candlelighters is a national organization with local chapters for parents of children with cancer. Mutual emotional support, education and stimulation and support for state and federal support for cancer research are the major objectives.

Make Today Count, Orville E. Kelly, Founder
P.O. Box 303
Burlington, Iowa 52601

This organization is dedicated to self-help for the cancer patient through the mutual support of fellow travelers in their journey with cancer.

Glossary of Cancer Terminology

ADENITIS: Inflammation of a gland.

ADENO: A prefix denoting relation to a gland or glands.

ADENOCARCINOMA: A carcinoma in which the cells are arranged in the form of glands; a malignant adenoma.

ADENOMA: Benign tumor, glandular in structure.

ADJUVANT THERAPY: A combination of surgery and chemotherapy and radiation therapy or a combination of any two of these modalities.

ALKYLATING AGENTS: A group of drugs that can be used to treat malignant diseases. These drugs change the shapes of important molecules, especially DNA, in rapidly growing cells.

ALOPECIA: Complete loss of hair.

AMINO ACID: One of the basic building blocks of protein.

ANEMIA: A deficiency in the quantity or quality of erythrocytes (red blood cells) in the circulating blood.

ANOREXIA: Lack or loss of appetite for food.

ANTIMETABOLITE: A chemical compound similar in structure to some essential substance of cell function. Some chemotherapeutic drugs are antimetabolites, effective in cancer therapy through their blocking of normal cell reaction.

APHASIA: Partial or complete inability to speak in an articulated manner or loss of verbal comprehension.

ASCITES: An accumulation of fluid in the peritoneal (abdominal) cavity.

BACTERIA: Very small one-celled organisms, most of which are harmless. Some of them, however, if they get into the human body can cause disease.

BENIGN: In describing a tumor, one which is relatively innocent.

BIOPSY: Excision of a small piece of tissue for microscopic examination.

BONE MARROW: Medulla or soft tissues in the hollow of long bones and in the extremities of long bones. All types of blood cells are made in the bone marrow.

BONE MARROW DEPRESSION: Damaged bone marrow.

BRONCHOGRAM: A roentgenogram of the lungs after the bronchi have been injected with opaque material.

CANCER: Any malignant tumor, made up chiefly of epithelial cells.

CARCINOGENIC: Producing cancer.

CARCINOMA: A malignant new growth made up of epithelial cells tending to infiltrate the surrounding tissue and give rise to mestastasis.

CANCER-IN-SITU: A lesion confined to the mucosal surface. No invasion or metastasis has occurred.

CACHEXIA: A condition of ill health, malnutrition and wasting.

CESIUM: A man-made radioactive substance used in radiation therapy.

CHEMOTHERAPY: The treatment of malignant disease by administering chemical compounds.

COBALT: One of the energy sources used in radiation therapy.

COLOSTOMY: The establishment of an artificial anus by making an opening into the colon.

CONSERVATIVE THERAPY: Aimed at the preservation of body integrity.

CORTISONE: A hormone of the adrenal cortex. It may be used in the treatment of some cancers.

CORDOTOMY: Surgical division of the spinal cord for relief of severe pain.

CURATIVE: Having a healing effect.

CYSTITIS: Inflammation of the bladder.

CYTOLOGY: The scientific study of cells, their origin, structure and function.

DESQUAMATION: Scaling of the skin or cuticle.

DIAGNOSIS: Recognition of disease states from symptoms, ausculation, inspection, palpation, percussion, posture, reflexes, general appearances, abnormalities, and abnormal attitudes and habits, microscopic and chemical examinations, x-rays.

DILATATION: 1. Expansion of an orifice with a dilator. 2. Expansion of an organ or vessel.

DNA: The chemical component of the genes which specifically directs the composition and function of the cell and is copied when a cell divides during growth. A mistake in the coding for particular proteins by the DNA may alter the function of that cell in the body.

DRUG: A medical substance used in the treatment of a disease.

DYSPHAGIA: Difficulty or pain occurring within 15 seconds of swallowing.

DYSPNEA: Difficult or labored breathing.

ERYTHROCYTES (RBC):   Carry oxygen to all parts of the body.

ETIOLOGY: The study of the causes of disease.

FATIGUE: Lassitude, tiredness, weariness.

FUNGUS: One-celled organism, most of which are harmless or even useful to humans (i.e. yeast). However, some fungi, if they get into the body can cause disease (i.e., pneumonia).

GLASS SLIDE: A small rectangular piece of clear glass on which material, such as blood or tissue, are placed on in order to look at them through a microscope.

GRANULOCYTES: A granular leukocyte or white blood cell (WBC). Function is to ward off germs and combat infections.

HEMATOCRIT: Volume of RBC per unit of circulating blood.

HEMATOLOGY: The scientific study of the blood.

HEMATURIA: Blood in the urine.

HEMAGLOBIN: The substance in RBC's that gives them their color and enables them to carry oxygen.

HEMOPTYSIS: Coughing up of blood.

HISTOLOGY: Study of the microscopic structure of tissue.

HORMONE: A chemical that is either produced by the body or man-made and normally helps keep the body functioning smoothly. Hormones are considered drugs when used in large amounts to treat certain diseases.

HYPODERMIC (HYPO):   Under the skin.

HOST: Person, animal, or plant harboring a disease organism or a neoplasm.

HYSTERECTOMY: Removal of the uterus.

ILEOSTOMY: An opening in the abdomen through which body wastes are discharged. The end portion of the ileum is brought through the abdominal wall to form a stoma.

INFECTION: When small organisms (such as bacteria, fungi, or viruses) enter the body and cause disease.

INFUSION: Introduction of a liquid into a vein.

INTRACAVITY: Into the body cavity.

INTRALESION: Into the lesion.

INTRAMUSCULAR: Into the muscle.

INTRATHECAL: In the spinal column.

INTRAVENOUS: Into the vein.

ISOTOPE: A radioactive member of a family of molecules.

JAUNDICE: A condition marked by yellow skin and eye whites, due to changes in the liver cells or obstructions, which cause the bile pigment, bilirubin, to be diffused into the blood.

LAETRILE: Unproven anti-cancer substance (remedy) derived from certain fruit kernels.

LAPAROTOMY: Abdominal incision for any operation on internal organs.

LAMINAR AIR FLOW ROOM: A private room provided for leukemia patients in an effort to shield them from environmental organisms through a specifically controlled atmosphere. Curtains of air sweep from the patient to the door as a part of the reverse isolation practiced.

LESION: A site of structural or functional change in body tissue produced by disease.

LEUKEMIA: Disease characterized by a great excess of white corpuscles.

LEUKOCYTES: WBC's which resist and combat infections.

LYMPH NODE: Gland that produces and stores white blood corpuscles and acts as a filter to keep harmful substances out of the system.

LINEAR ACCELERATOR: Acceleration of an electron in a straight line.

MALAISE: Discomfort, uneasiness, indisposition, often indicative of infection.

MALIGNANT: Dangerous or a threat to life. A malignant tumor has the capacity for destructive invasion of surrounding tissue and for metastasis.

MAMMOGRAPHY: An x-ray of the breast.

METASTASIS: A new focus of tumor growth started by spread of malignant cells from the primary site to a new location in the body.

MUCOSITIS: Redness or soreness of the lining of the mouth, throat, or vagina.

NAUSEA: Inclination to vomit.

NECROSIS: Death of areas of tissue or bone surrounded by healthy parts.

NEOPLASM: Any new and abnormal growth such as a tumor.

ONCOLOGY: The study of all aspects of malignant disease.

PALLIATION: Temporary relief.

PALPABLE: Perceptible by touch.

PALPITATION: Rapid, violent or throbbing pulsation, as an abnormally rapid, throbbing or fluttering of the heart.

PAPANOCOLAOU SMEAR (PAP TEST):   A method of collecting and staining cells to diagnose cancer.

PATHOLOGY: The study of disease or disease processes.

PLACEBO: An inactive substance or preparation; any effect attributed to a pill, potion, or procedure, but not to its pharmacodynomic or specific properties.

PLATELETS: Derived from giant bone marrow cells. They are pale discs found in normal blood and aid in coagulation.

PROSTATECTOMY: Excision of part or all of the prostate gland.

PRURITUS: Severe itching.

RADIATION: Treatment with a radioactive substance.

RADIOTHERAPY: The treatment of a disease by application of roentgen rays, radium, ultraviolet and other radiations.

REMISSION: A period of time in the treatment of cancer when the symptoms have abated.

RESECTION: Partial excision.

RBC (ERYTHROCYTES):   Carry oxygen to all parts of the body.

SCARIFICATION: To scratch the skin or make numerous small incisions on the skin.

SARCOMA: A cancer arising in connective tissue.

SCAN: After administration of a drug containing a minute amount of radioactive substance a geiger counter machine with camera traces the concentration of radioactive substance and outlines the organ.

SIMULATE: Treatment planning where an x-ray is taken of the treatment area with an x-ray machine that imitates the treatment machine. The exact area to be treated is marked.

SPINAL PUNCTURE: Puncture of the spinal cavity, with a needle, to extract spinal fluid.

STAGING: Determining period in the course of disease.

STOMA: An opening on a body surface, surgically constructed. Example: colostomy, laryngectomy, or urinary ostomy.

STOMATITIS: Redness and soreness of stoma.

SUPPOSITORY: Medication inserted rectally.

SUSCEPTIBLE: Having little resistance to a disease.

SYNDROME: A set of symptoms which occur together.

THROMBOCYTES (PLATELETS): Derived from giant bone marrow cells. They are pale discs found in normal blood and aid in coagulation.

THROMBOCYTOPENIA: Abnormal decrease in the number of blood platelets.

TOMOGRAM: An x-ray taken at the depth of interest. One with a special machine, it blurs out unwanted areas.

TOXICITY: The condition of being poisonous.

TRANSFUSION: Injection of the blood of one person into the blood vessels of another.

TUMOR: An abnormal swelling or enlargement, either benign or malignant.

URINALYSIS: Analysis of the urine.

WBC (LEUKOCYTES): Resist and combat infections.

X-RAY: A photograph obtained by use of x-rays.

ULTRASOUND SCANNER: A machine which directs radiowaves through the body; the wave bounces back and shows an outline of the internal organs.

GLOSSARY REFERENCES

Josephine K. Craytor & Margot L. Fass. *The Nurse and the Cancer Patient.* Lippincott, 1972.

Baker, Roland & Gilchrist. *You and Leukemia.* Mayo Comprehensive Cancer Center. Rochester, Minnesota. November 1976.

T. J. Deeley, E. J. Fisk, M. A. Gough. *A Guide to Oncological Nursing.* Edinburgh and London: Churchill Livingstone, 1974.

A Cancer Source Book for Nurses. American Cancer Society, 1975.

Tobers Cyclopedic Medical Dictionary. T. A. Davis Company.

Suggested Reading

Abrams, Ruth D., M.S. *Not Alone With Cancer:* Springfield, IL: Charles C. Thomas, 1974.

    Ruth Abrams has been working with cancer patients and their families for more than twenty years. Her book is a sensitive and practical guide for families of patients with cancer.

James, Muriel, Jongeword, Dorothy, *Born to Win: Transactional Analysis with Gestalt Experiments.* Menlo Park, CA: Addison-Wesley, 1971.

    This book is especially helpful in understanding and developing skills in interpersonal relationships.

Kelly, Orville E., *Make Today Count:* New York: Delacorte, 1975.

    An autobiographical account of how one man found new meaning in life as a result of cancer, and through his experience is helping thousands of fellow patients around the world.

Weatherhead, Leslie D., *The Christian Agnostic.* Nashville: Abingdon, 1975.

    A noted clergyman's journey through doubt to faith.

Baker, Lynne S., *You and Leukemia, A Day at a Time*. Rochester, MN: Mayo Comprehensive Cancer Center, 1976.

"Childhood Leukemia: A Pamphlet for Parents," U.S. Department of Health, Education and Welfare, National Cancer Institute, Bethesda, Maryland 20014.

Progress Against Leukemia, U. S. Department of Health and Welfare, National Cancer Institute, Bethesda, Maryland 20014.

Sherman, Mikie, *Feeding the Sick Child*, Department of Health and Welfare, National Cancer Institute, Bethesda, Maryland 20014.

Sherman, Mikie, *The Leukemic Child*, Department of Health and Welfare, National Cancer Institute, Bethesda, Maryland 20014.